MEDUSA'S CLOT

THE ILL-HUMOR OF PULMONARY EMBOLISM

DR. MICHAEL D. HELZNER

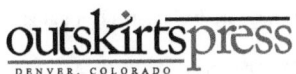
outskirtspress
DENVER, COLORADO

Dedication:

To my wife Cassandra, you are my every breath drawn.

To my children Cynthia and Alexander, one day I hope to grow up to be just like you.

To my spine specialist Dr. Guy Lee for always having my back.

Human beings will continue to measure the intrinsic worth of things whether they be objects or concepts with the utmost exactness, and will persist in doing so rather imprecisely.

M. D. Helzner D.O.

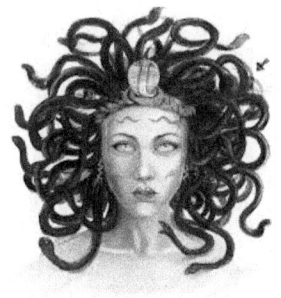

Contents

INTRODUCTION : NUMBERS

THE MONSTER THAT GOOGLE OMITTED

In 1818 author Mary Shelley wrote in Frankenstein "I will glut the maw of death, until it is satiated with the blood of your remaining friends." What do we really perceive about the disease known as pulmonary embolism that by some statistical measures as proffered by the Centers for Disease Control and Prevention may affect 300,000-600,000 people per year and glut the maw of death with 60,000-100,000 American lives per year? And that may be understated.

That is about 2 patients per 1000 and if you are lucky enough to become an octogenarian that number devolves into 1 out of 100. During 2007-2009, there was an estimated annual average 547,596 adult hospitalizations for venous thromboembolism. An estimated 348,558 had a diagnosis of deep vein thrombosis which is the entity most responsible for the pulmonary catastrophe. During the same time period an approximately 277,549 had a diagnosis of pulmonary embolism. Roughly 78,511 of the adult hospitalizations had both. A 1991 study done in

Worchester, Massachusetts concluded that more than half the cases of venous thrombo-embolic disease are never diagnosed. If one is with child the risk is 4-5 fold and so it remains after the mother delivers that bundle of joy for a number of months. In fact pulmonary embolism is one of the leading causes of maternal death in the Western world. Even if not pregnant the odds of having an embolism is higher than a male counterpart and if Afro-American it is even worse. It can according to some non-governmental sources purportedly kill over 100,000 of us yearly. Up to 30% within a month of the draconian diagnosis. In the fraction of a second it takes to Google "The clot in my lung,"10- 25% can die before the web page is finished loading and that is with a relatively speedy Wi-Fi connection. If one is unfortunate enough to have one and yet fortunate enough to survive then there is a 1 in 3 chance of experiencing yet another in the decade that ensues. Mark your smart phone's calendar.

Even if one is young and in great athletic shape protection is not bestowed. In fact the sportsperson may be in an increased risk category to develop a clot. Athletes often get dehydrated, they are constantly travelling for long periods of time, there are injuries to the lower extremities, and they occasionally need to get their knee or hip operated on. Add a slow resting pulse that makes red blood cells sluggish and a coagulum may form before the next contest. These are just five hazards. There are others.

It was dubbed the "Economy Class Syndrome" but a clot enjoys 1st class too despite the wider seats and extra leg room. If older, on certain medicines, mildly obese, have a gene mutation, or sit near a window seat where one tends not to move about the peril increases.

Most pulmonary embolisms are in the inchoate phase a clot lodged in the deep veins of the legs called a deep vein thrombosis. Ever hear of this killer? I am not surprised only about 1 in 4 Americans have. They can in reality originate from any vein or even the heart but the overall majority get their start below the belly-button. It is estimated that there are over 2 million new cases a year of these southern confederate trouble makers. 34% of people who develop what is known as deep vein thrombosis will have life-long complications such as painful swelling, pruritus (itching), ulcerations, discoloration, and scaling of the affected limb. Among patients with a leg clot who did not wear compression stockings 20-82% developed these issues recognized as post-thrombotic syndrome. A devastating sequel but some others are infinitely worse.

It is estimated that 5-8% of the U.S. population have a genetic mutation that increases the chance for abnormal clotting 3-5 times. The overall majority of these people have absolutely no idea that they are literally sitting on a powder keg. If the 8% is accurate then we are dealing with the same number of people who have diabetes mellitus in the United States. Over 25 million. Fortunately most will not develop a pulmonary embolism/deep vein thrombosis but I advance in supposition only that with certain life style decisions the potential for something bad increases markedly and the most recent studies are substantiating that supposition. A female's choice of contraception or the decision to go on estrogen replacement therapy for those post-menopausal hot flashes can begin a game of Russian roulette. A male's choice to go on testosterone, an occupation that keeps one firmly sitting without respite, and the weekend mesmerized casino player adds bullets to the chamber.

Over two millennium ago it was the Greek mathematician Euclid who averred "That Life is written in the number." Let us see as to what "The Father of Geometry" was referring.

To put things in perspective simply enter onto your computer's search engine "Leading causes of deaths in the United States" and this is what the Internet furnishes based on the reporting year 2013 from the Centers for Disease Control(CDC). The 10 least wanted hits are what follows:

1) Heart disease 611,105
2) Cancer 584,881.
3) Chronic Lower respiratory diseases 149,205.
4) Accidents 130,557 (Accidents and stroke have recently flip-flopped. Texting perhaps?)
5) Stroke 128,978
6) Alzheimer's 84,767
7) Diabetes 75,578
8) Influenza and pneumonia 56,979
9) Kidney Disease 47,112
10) Suicide 41,149

I am unsure why pulmonary embolism is the (I don't get any respect) Rodney Dangerfield of lethal diseases but it is distressing to see it, or should I say not see it. In essence pulmonary embolism should be #6 or #7. Unlike the old analog world where people received their information from multiple sources, today if it is not found on Google it does not exist. I am unsure if it is a miscalculation or a form of algorithm negligence but I do not believe it is purposeful. Nevertheless it is hard to look at the staggering statistics as it is hard not to and cast them aside. In the United States and the United Kingdom if one adds up the annual deaths from prostate cancer, HIV, and breast cancer, the combination is second to those dying from pulmonary embolism. I assume not all algorithms are created equally but it is the 3rd leading cause of cardiovascular death in the United States as it is simultaneously the 3rd leading cause of death in our nation's infirmaries. Despite the prevalence most cases are not recognized ante mortem (prior to death), and less than 10% of patients who died from a pulmonary embolism (PE) ever received any treatment.

From 1969-2013 death rates from heart disease, cancer, strokes, accidents, and diabetes have all dropped. The death rate from COPD (chronic obstructive pulmonary disease) during the same time interval has increased. The data suggests that the death rate from pulmonary embolism has sadly done the same and in stealthy fashion.

If one goes to different websites there are disparate numbers, but even if the lower estimates are accepted the somber fact remains that they are truly mind-boggling. Certainly if the self-deprecating comedian Dangerfield was alive today there would no doubt be a joke about "Clots of Fun."

In the real world this is no laughing matter. It is one of this nation's biggest yet least known healthcare headaches. Ironically it is associated with migraines.

Plainly I am not alone in my beliefs. In a 2003 article entitled "Embolism:" Part I by Samuel Goldhaber, M.D. and C Elliot M.D the authors early on state after citing some statistics, "This makes pulmonary embolism possibly as deadly as an illness as acute myocardial infarction (heart attack). Nevertheless, the lay public has not been well educated about PE (pulmonary embolism)." The National Blood Clot Alliance did a recent survey that showed nearly 80% of the general public is not aware of the life-threatening blood clot risk called deep vein thrombosis.

Not just the lay public, I recently had a long conversation with an experienced ICU (intensive care unit) nurse who had a pulmonary embolism in August of 2014. We literally played 20 questions. She was exhausted and could not understand why? What should she be doing going forward? Why did she have one? Was an intravenous filter required? Should she be wearing compression stockings? Did she have a genetic proclivity? What could she do to avoid another? Do her children need testing? I cannot remember the other 12 questions.

I have tried to develop a workable hypothesis as to why the deep vein thrombosis remains relatively recondite. I think one of the most common, most worn out, and yet most true phrases in the world is "It is probably a combination of things" followed by "It is what it is." There is yet to be discovered in the discipline of physics a unified field theory. Basically a theory that combines the universe's fundamental forces and elementary particles in terms of a single field. Albert Einstein went to his grave in 1955 after an abdominal aortic aneurysm (ballooning) ruptured. With all his accomplishments he died crestfallen unable to prove that which he believe existed. I, born in 1955 at Albert Einstein Hospital in Philadelphia certainly have not stumbled upon an integrative reason for the evasive clot in the" un-discipline" of medicine. An unfolding genius I was not nor ever would be.

That being averred I was thinking about my days as a medical student which led me to a hunch and it is only a partial one. I remember quite vividly attending lectures in cardiology (study of the heart) given by the cardiologist (heart doctor), pulmonology (study of the lungs) given by the pulmonologist (lung doctor), endocrinology (study of hormones) given by the endocrinologist (hormone doctor), gastroenterology (study of the gastrointestinal tract) given by the gastroenterologist, and so on down the line. I remember the names of all the lecturers from over 35 years ago, yet I cannot recall any specific lectures on the peripheral circulatory system which is the system of veins and arteries in the arms and legs. Often with the major organ systems these germane arteries and veins were discussed only then. There is yet another phantom transport system called the lymphatic system that is even more mysterious and abstruse. The point is there are no vein-ologists, arterial-ologist, or lymph-ologists.

I recall as a callow intern the attending physician would need to consult cardiology, hematology, and etc. but when a patient had swollen ankles or decreased peripheral pulses, he or she would order a vascular consult, no 'ology'. There was one healer who would ambulate mysteriously around the hospital with a device called a Doppler (ultrasound) and take some measurements. I was never really sure what his training was. He was not a surgeon. Did he do an internal medicine residency first and then sub-specialized? Vascular specialists today are usually surgeons and tend to work more on the arterial side of hospitalized patients. Although recently much is being done with varicose veins and refluxing venous valves. Arteries with few exceptions contain blood that is rich in oxygen. Venous blood in general is lower in oxygen.

Medicine can be confusing in as much as it is basically divided among medical specialties and surgical specialties with crossovers. If a cardiologist thinks heart surgery is required then a referral to a heart surgeon is made, unless the surgery can be done with catheters and then one might be referred to an interventional cardiologist. If an endocrinologist thinks a thyroid needs removal then a referral to a thyroid surgeon is prescribed, but the endocrinologist can perform a "surgical" procedure to biopsy the thyroid. If a neurologist thinks one needs spine surgery the patient will be referred to a neurosurgeon or an orthopedic surgeon who sub-specializes in spine procedures. If a patient has chronic sinusitis then he or she may be referred to an

ENT doctor whose specialty is called o-to-rhin-o-lar-yn-gol-o-gy. They can treat the sinuses medically or surgically. Quite a nine syllabized mouthful for a specialty that operates all over the face but rarely in the mouth unless accompanied by an oral-maxillary surgeon, who is in fact a dentist. Some surgeries like a nose job can be done by ENT or plastic surgeons. Some skin issues can be treated by a dermatologist or someone in the field of plastics. Other physicians have taken some additional training and can do aesthetic surgery like hair replacement or getting rid of those unsightly superficial spider veins. Endovascular (inside the vein or artery) surgery can now be performed by a dizzying array of physicians such as radiologists, neurologists, neurosurgeons, cardiologists, cardiovascular surgeons, and vascular surgeons.

It seems that if an individual has an issue with a "target organ" it is easy to find out as to whom to visit. But if there is a problem with the network that carries oxygen to and from these organs one may have a problem as to where to go. This seems particularly true if the problem involves the veins.

I called three institutions and relayed to the operator that I was a patient with vein issues and wanted to see a specialist. I was in all three cases directed to the hospital's vascular lab. It is a lab not a doctor's office. Additionally most patients would not be able to discern that the problem is with their venous system anyway. They just might be experiencing an ache in the calf or see some lower leg swelling.

So maybe the human cognizance has an easier time categorizing solid organ systems than the vast and diffuse connecting transportation networks, and thus is more in tune to their pathologies. If things can be neatly categorized they are easier to remember and if the human brain can recollect something more easily then possibly one inherently becomes more aware. If a passenger was to take a train ride across Western Europe and keep a diary probably few of journal entries would be about the train tracks in Spain, France, or Germany. Humans appear somewhat conduit challenged. I think this is so because evolution seems more predicated on object recognition and endpoints (food, water, sex, and shelter) then travel routes.

The patient will probably first see their primary care provider who could be a physician, nurse practitioner, or physician assistant. Assuming the diagnosis is made and it is not often obvious, the patient will be referred out. If a deep vein thrombosis is suspected then the referral should be made to the emergency room because 5- 10% of the time the thrombosis (clot) will travel to the lungs and lethally tamper with them.

Watch television long enough and there are commercials for breast cancer, diabetes, high cholesterol, erectile dysfunction, atrial fibrillation, stroke, autism, Alzheimer's disease, heart attack, arthritis, prostate cancer, alcohol and drug abuse, acne, baldness, HPV, shingles, flu, ALS, muscular dystrophy, asthma, gastrointestinal reflux, arthritis, hearing loss, and weight gain. These are just part of the "Breaking Bad" punchbowl marathon. Venous thromboembolism does not even get an honorable mention. How dishonorable is this screeching absurdity.

Take a casual ride on the metropolitan area's expressways and there are billboards boasting Voted best in cancer; Best in orthopedics; Best in cardiac care; Best in stroke care; and Best in rehabilitation. All from some of the finest institutions in this sovereignty who for some reason blot out the clot from their advertising budget.

The irony is that if an individual stays on the highway or watches the TV long enough and does not move from the seat for a couple of hours, chances of getting a thrombus in the legs increase. If that clot decides to take a little trip it does so by heading north on the anatomy's bloody Venous Highway. It enters the heart's right atrium (upper chamber), sight-sees the right ventricle (lower chamber) for a fugacious period of time and then after being turbo-charged backpacks and then lodges snuggly into one or more arteries of the lungs. Trust me it is a most disagreeable passenger and a worse houseguest as he often brings other family members. If the clot burden is sizable enough the last thing the eyes may ever see on this earth is a commercial for the seemingly ubiquitous "Low T (testosterone) Syndrome." As paradox would have it the male hormone is associated with the same embolism that just killed the viewer and put him in that T-shaped coffin.

To be fair the golden-voiced announcer did mention the side effects but one would have to set the DVR speed to "slow" in order to hear and process it. Just when the lounger thought watching television with its parental controls was safe there is paronomasically speaking a "remote" possibility that it is anything but.

I am writing this book because the subject is quite figuratively and literally close to my heart. Twice in fact. One small pulmonary embolism in 2006 after one of my spine surgeries and one that was rather large accompanied by another small one in 2013. The second embolism came after playing blackjack with legs crossed at a gambling hall for a ridiculous amount of time hoping to win the "big one." I guess I did or at least the right lower lobe of my lung did. Counting the cards and not the hours is a losing strategy. I will go into more detail later in this book.

As a physician I have made every effort to present this subject in a clear fashion to the non-medical segments of the population. It is a complex subject and there is at times a scintilla of science that must make a few cameo appearances. Let me apologize in advance. After my second pulmonary embolism I am no longer longwinded. Perhaps my loss is the reader's gain?

After nearly thirty-five previous surgical procedures I can state unequivocally that nothing has had a more profound effect on my mental, spiritual, and physical being than this disease. Actually that last statement is only 1/3 true and thus not unequivocally. In 1987 my daughter had an ischemic (deprived of oxygen) event to her brainstem, coded, and needed cardiopulmonary resuscitation (CPR). It was that event that unhinged my mental and spiritual instrumentation. That consequence of which will become more clear in chapter 13. I have not recovered from either

1987 or 2013.

Penultimately I hope this small book will in some small way impact the need to take this disease more seriously. It is bad enough that such a potentially lethal disease remains on the perimeter. It is patently egregious that it remains on the periphery of that perimeter. The vitiated state of things will only change with education, allocated financial resources, and awareness. This is a major public health problem in the United States whose many deaths can be prevented.

Finally it is my fervent desideratum that venous thromboembolism smartly abbreviated as VTE which is the sobriquet for the fraternal twins of pulmonary embolism (PE) and deep vein thrombosis (DVT) is soon included on the Googled "The 10 Least Wanted List" and that one day it ultimately isn't.

Enjoy "Medusa's Clot" but not at one time, not without getting up intermittently and getting the blood to circulate in your legs a bit. Sitting is the new smoking they say. The statistics quantitatively may be disparate, but with a pulmonary embolism your life is taken down a few notches. Or possibly all of them.

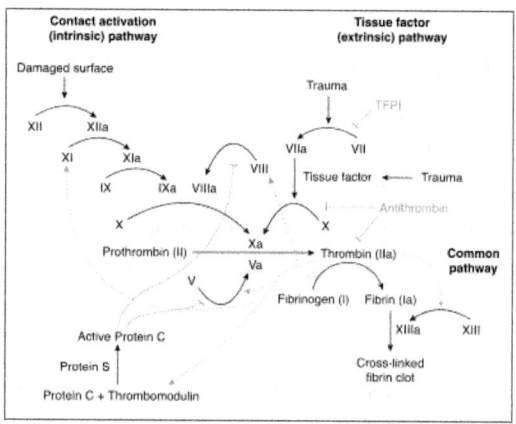

FIGURE 1. CLOT FORMATION.

PLEASE DO NOT WORRY ABOUT THE FUZZY DIAGRAM ABOVE.

GENESIS: THE COAGULATION CASCADE and THE THROMBUS AMONG US

THOSE WHO MAY BE more curious may want to refer to Figure 1 online. It is neither necessary nor sufficient to cause any concern. It is called the coagulation cascade where the story begins.

A thrombus is simply the medical term for clot and will hitherto be the designation intermittently going forward. A thrombosis is when a thrombus obstructs the blood flow in a circulatory vessel. In this book we are dealing with those that for the most part are formed in the torso's lower veins but they can have other origins.

Another term we need to define is embolism which is any detached intravascular (inside the blood vessel) mass. This could be in the form of a gas, solid, or liquid that is capable of creating a vessel blockage away from its point of origin.

Though we will be dealing solely with thromboembolism, which is one made of blood clots, there are many others. Some examples are fat embolism, tumor embolism, parasitic egg embolism, cholesterol embolism, air embolism, septic embolism, tissue embolism, foreign body embolism, and what I have always found most intriguing, an amniotic fluid embolism. Each one is associated with certain clinical situations. The latter might actually contain fetal cells, hair, or other debris that enters the pregnant mother's bloodstream via the placenta.

Closely related to the amniotic fluid embolism is the air embolism that has several diverse causes such as an accidental or purposeful intravenous injection of air, surgical procedures, lung trauma, bomb/explosive injuries, scuba diving, and a rather unique etiology that involves a certain sexual activity performed on a pregnant woman. Without getting graphic the vaginal vault can accommodate up to a liter of air. That air volume can strip the amniotic membranes away from the uterus and pass into the mother's venous circulation. Like all of its cousins the air embolism in bubble form travels through the large vein draining the lower half of the body known as the inferior vena cava (IVC) and lodges into one or more pulmonary arteries. If the mother is even more unlucky and has a certain heart defect the globules can enter the mother's brain with fatal consequences.

It is important to realize that a thrombus does not exist in a vacuum. It can be a best friend or a worst enemy depending on the situation. It is the end product of a complex sequence of biochemical and physiological reactions. Platelets also known as thrombocytes are those pesky short-lived first responders that initially rush to patch a breach in a vessel wall. I have "seen" them plenty of times while shaving carelessly. They circulate in the vital fluid of all mammals and when activated stick together to form a temporary plug until the" navy seals" of coagulation (diagram above) reinforce the plug with a glue made up of primarily fibrin (a protein) threads. It is important for the reader to recognize that the coagulation cascade is so much more infinitely complicated and along with these coagulation factors there are cofactors and regulators molecularly hovering about in their respective intrinsic, extrinsic, and common pathways. Some of them are present to prevent clotting from getting out of hand.

In the end if everything goes exactly to plan there is a fibrin patch preventing one from hemorrhaging.

These "navy seals" are in reality proteins that are portrayed as Roman numerals but they also have names. Perhaps a little intimacy with these creatures won't hurt.

I Fibrinogen
II Prothrombin
III Tissue Factor
IV Calcium
V Labile Factor
VI UNASSIGNED
VII Stable Factor
VIII Antihemophilic Factor A

IX Antihemophilic Factor B (Christmas factor-named after the patient Stephen Christmas who had hemophilia B)

X Stuart-Power Factor

XI Thromboplastin antecedent

XII Hageman Factor

XIII Fibrin- Stabilizing Factor

In medical school because there is so much rote memorization especially in the first two years, classical mnemonics have been handed down from generation to generation as well as ongoing newer piquant ones to help the student remember. There are so many mnemonics that I tried to invent a mnemonic to not only remind myself how to spell mnemonic but to remember the list of mnemonics. I was woefully unsuccessful at both endeavors.

One of the classics is a method to recall the 12 human cranial nerves which are also notated in Roman numerals. They are seen below. That empire surely left its mark! I was taught this one. "Oh Oh Oh To Touch And Feel Virgin Girls' Vaginas And Hymen." There are many variants and I think the religious in the class probably used one less ribald but every bit as effective. They are as follows.

I Olfactory: OH

II Optic: OH

III Oculomotor: OH

IV Trochlear: TO

V Trigeminal: TOUCH

VI Abducens: AND

VII Facial: FEEL

VIII Vestibulocochlear: VIRGIN
IX Glossopharyngeal: GIRLS'
X Vagus: VAGINAS
XI Accessory: AND
XII Hypoglossal: HYMEN

For those interested in impressing one's friends with the aforementioned coagulation factors, this ditty has gained popularity. A person just has to remember that there is no longer a factor VI (left over from bygone days) and factor XI is a stepchild. "Foolish People Try Climbing Long Slopes After Christmas, Some Have Fallen." The real reason why I took the time to name them is that when we discuss certain genetic mutations, there are some often identified by their names not their numeral.

If one wakes up one morning and one's nose is profusely bleeding, a thrombus is what one should hope for. If a person is having a heart attack or a certain type of stroke one would want just about anything else. The human body when it is exquisitely firing on all cylinders is able to modulate between excess bleeding and excess clotting. Like the macroscopic world external to us our inner microscopic universe is also underwritten in a binary narrative (black-white, yes-no, on-off). When we get too hot we sweat to dissipate heat, when we get too cold we shiver to produce warmth. When we are active our hearts speed up so hemoglobin can carry more oxygen to our tissues and when we relax the cordiform organ slows down. Living organisms have developed an uncanny system of ostensibly infinite evolutionary homeostatic checks and balances.

But there are imperfections and because it is so efficient a system that when things are just a bit off the results can be devastating as there is little room for error.

Not everything in our constitution is that unforgiving and affords us some well-deserved slack. Our blood pressure for example can go from very low to very high and one may be totally asymptomatic until it hits critical levels. The pulmonary vascular system which has two arterial supplies (most organs have one) is remarkably accommodating to volume and flow. Microscopic processes are more finely tuned.

So why do things go askew? Because the state of being is simply a complex rigged game that commences soon after our mommies and daddies conceive us. Often on a Saturday night after dinner and a movie but before the hebdomadal monologue on Saturday Night Live. At that moment of conception a molecular lottery begins defining us in every which way throughout our lives. Even if we are lucky, it is only in a relative sense. We lose 6.5% of lean muscle mass every decade after age 30, arthritis ensues, our cognition decreases as our cerebral endowments become less elastic, our immune system assumes the form of a sleepy and less vigilant bodyguard, the waistline grows closer to our car's steering wheel while our hairline recedes towards its headrest. Sables, Jaguars, Mustangs-Oh my! Our arteries narrow along with our worldviews and we have a more difficult time SEEING that we have developed a HEARING loss as calcium relentlessly escapes from our skeletons. The sexual drive reduces its gear as the vagina contracts, the mammary glands droop, the testicles shrink, and the prostate expands. The once optimistic penis takes on the appearance of an antiquated Jewish comedian performing at the Catskills Mountains. Dr. Pangloss-stein looked rather funny even when he was younger. Our senses though dulled cannot help but to notice the denouement. Happy birthday y'all! The list marches on unfettered as time merely indulges us. Ultimately we all lose and to this day despite a very sentient spiritual peregrination I highly doubt that there is an overtime period after quietus.

When bad things happen to us we usually query "Why me?" Realistically what is preventing the cosmos from replying "Why not you?" "Why should things go right all the time or at any time?" There is an inherent entropy in the world where we reside both microscopically and macroscopically. Dr. Richard Dawkins, the brilliant biologist when discussing mutations likens it to when we are making many duplicates on a copy machine and there is the occasional paper that emerges crumpled or cock-eyed. When copying this tome page 96 came out essentially shredded. Similar to what most publishers did to my original manuscript. Ironically page 96 was ensconced in the chapter discussing genes and their mutations. Also Dr. Dawkins looks at us as a product not as an immutable blue print but as a recipe with minute variations. In another words not all cakes that are baked following the same set of instructions taste or even look the same. One can get a haircut by the same stylist every four weeks at exactly noon and assuredly the amount of bristles cut, their lengths, and amount of mousse applied will vary month to month. I know with my barber I often leave his establishment looking like a character from Shakespeare's "Hamlet." A decent haircut "Perchance to dream!"

A pulmonary thrombotic embolism cannot exist without a premonitory thrombus. That thrombus can form in any vein or even in the heart but most of the time trouble begins in the deep veins of the calf. It is commonly dubbed a deep vein thrombosis sensibly abbreviated as DVT. Most thrombi in the calf veins do not migrate to the lungs but around 20% of them will propagate proximally into the deep veins of the thigh and once there 50-60% of those thrombi head towards the pulmonary vessels many in an unforthcoming fashion producing no declarations. At least 50% of DVTs are asymptomatic. When they do produce symptoms the calf is often swollen, warm, and painful. The condition is called phlebitis.

Before we take leave of the thrombus among us and its associated trouble making thrombosis it is important to know that the deep veins of the legs do not have a monopoly on them as previously alluded to. In clinical medicine they are found in such varied places as veins of the liver, kidney, neck, upper extremities, abdomen, and brain. To make matters worse they also form in arteries supplying blood to our viscera (internal organs) and cause ischemia (lack of oxygen). Behind many strokes and heart attacks is the arterial thrombosis. People inflicted with sickle cell disease and trait often have a coagulation cascade gone wild. A major thrombosis to the arteries of the legs can cause gangrene to set in rather quickly. One to the kidney and it can be rendered totally non-functional.

A particular malady affecting the pregnant or women who just delivered is the HELLP syndrome. It is an acronym that stands for Hemolysis (red blood cells breaking), Elevated Liver enzymes, & Low Platelets. It is an affliction that is related to preeclampsia where the mother's blood pressure goes up and abnormal amounts of protein enter the urine. Strokes, seizures, kidney failure, and excessive bleeding can all follow.

Some 48,000 women will develop the HELLP syndrome annually and if not caught early there is a high death rate for both mother and child. What is the proposed mechanism? Apparently it all starts with the figure 1, the coagulation cascade. Fibrin being laid down in arteries act as a strainer for the erythrocytes (red blood cells) causing them to break up and a disaster ensues.

The thrombus among us at times can morph into a creature best avoided. One tiny genetic misread and one's essence and existence might be defined by excessive clotting or bleeding. Sometimes the imbalanced dualism can coexist but rarely cogently. It is similar to when one first awakens prior to any act of pandiculation loathing the idea of entering the shower and then once in, abhors leaving it.

CHAPTER II

DEUTERONOMY "FROM GOD DOWN to the STONES"

BY THE TIME most of us have graduated high school the names Albert Einstein, Sir Isaac Newton, Charles Darwin, Louis Pasteur, Benjamin Franklin, and Thomas Edison have been introduced. All quintessential multi-faceted geniuses that are born at the approximate rate of 1 per 300,000 live births, at least by some crazy statistician's analysis. Does Leonardo even need a surname to be recognized as the man from Vinci? There were many more unsung who got their "nerd on."

Many of these characters were replete with psychiatric issues and eccentricities. Mozart when he was not composing a symphony or opera often made crazy and puerile scatological epistolary references. Did the stylistic wunderkind have an anal fixation? Michelangelo was more often than not cheerless and somber. Researchers today believe he was a high functioning autistic. Thomas Jefferson prone to bouts of depression and migraines brought on by stress had many gifts including the ability to rationalize on the drop of a dime. His depiction would not be on the American nickel till 1938. Vincent van Gogh was plagued by mental illness his whole life, possibly borderline personality disorder. He committed suicide in 1890. Darwin seemed to have OCD (obsessive compulsive disorder) and hypochondriasis (health anxiety). Napoleon among his other "short" comings had well a Napoleonic complex (a pejorative social stereotype). Famous people often become so because of a magnificent gene package embroidered with the ribbon of hard work. This box is often costly. Many would have benefitted by having a psychiatrist on speed dial. To the age old question does history make people or do people make history, I tend to give the slight edge to the latter.

If I may let me introduce a genius who appeared remarkably balanced, normal, and without a severely atrophied emotional IQ. Dr. Rudolf Carl Virchow, physician, pathologist, biologist, esteemed public health advocate, egalitarian social democrat, and cosmopolitan writer. In high school he announced that he wanted to "acquire an all-round knowledge of nature-from G-d down to the stones." History has surely affirmed that the professor did procure his goal.

At age 71 he was awarded the prestigious Copley

Medal in 1892 given yearly by the London's Royal Society. Early on he studied science and medicine at the Prussian Military Academy on scholarship of course. Enlightened by viewpoints emanating from both France and England he developed a wide *Weltanschauung* (worldview) different than his somewhat stodgy coevals in Berlin.

As chair of pathological anatomy at the University of Wurzburg beginning in 1849 he concentrated on venous thrombosis and cell theory. Along the way to his ground breaking work he was outwardly the first to recognize the cells associated with leukemia and pioneered the standard procedure of autopsy including the liver probe used to take the temperature of a carcass. One may appreciate that fact next time the hit TV series CSI is broadcasted.

Furthermore his studies on the human cranium (phrenology) in 1885 contradicted the then questionable science supporting racism. Needless to say the Aryan Race superiority advocates were not pleased. An epigone named Adolph Hitler would be born 4 years later. The mustached misanthrope would eventually find fault with Rudolph's scientific findings many years before the paltry skirmish of World War II.

Virchow was an ardent supporter of full and unlimited democracy, education, freedom, and unfettered prosperity which were antipodal to the then German political powers. They were in the midst of the revolutionary tumult engulfing Europe. National Socialism and Communism were still in-utero at the time but growing along with the primal cries of global liberalism. Still dominant however were Prussian militarism and Machiavellian monarchies along with their glistening bayonets and flourishing sabers. Republicanism in Europe embraced by Virchow was still a long way off as was cultural humility.

The professor was a man way ahead of his time. He angered cherub-Chancellor/Prime Minister Otto von Bismarck so badly by criticizing his bloated military budget that the statesman invited the scientist to a duel. Apocryphally recorded as the "Sausage Duel," Virchow was challenged and thus was able to choose the weapons. The doctor offered Bismarck a link of sausage infected with the parasite Trichinella spiralis. Evidently the Chancellor was not ready to say auf Wiedersehen and incontestably removed himself from the food fight. The bellicose and snobbish Bismarck needed to diet anyway and later on the two worked together to curtail the strength and political influence of the Catholic Church.

There is no dearth of medical terminology named after our sage and hero. In fact there are 15 items with his attached appellation. Thirteen of which are rather arcane. It would stretch credulity to think that anyone would be informed of them off the top of their craniums. The two that all good medical students should appreciate are Virchow's node and Virchow's triad.

Virchow's node is a physical finding of an enlarged lymph node (gland) above the left clavicle (collar bone) that may represent a gastrointestinal or pulmonary malignancy. Often there is a modicum of serendipity on its discovery. Virchow's triad is the 19th century eponymous model for venous thrombosis and embolism. To this day it remains so. Perhaps it is a bit ironic that the general public comprehends as much about this pioneering scientific legend and "Father of modern pathology" as the potentially lethal disease whose origins he figured out. He died in 1902 at the age of 80.

We now turn to Virchow's famous triad of venous stasis, trauma, and hypercoagulable states. Find a thrombosis and one will find at its source at least 1 of the aforementioned and often a combination.

When I was in medical school with Fred Flintstone and Barney Rubble DVT and PE were often treated as discrete related entities. In essence they are manifestations of the same disease process separated only by their locations. Imagine a train leaving Philadelphia and heading north to New York City. On arrival to the "Big Apple" the boxcar is essentially unchanged but for its location. Quantum physicists and erudite philosophers may disagree but to our everyday senses it is the same vehicle. The only thing that changed were the respective train stations analogous to the southern deep venous tracks of the leg and the northern arterial tracks of the lungs.

For many, about 10% it is indeed the terminus.

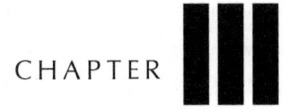

REVELATION
VIRCHOW'S TRIAD

STATING THE PROFESSOR'S triad is easy but now we need to take a look at these three factors more closely with what Virchow often used, a microscope.

1) Trauma is basically damage to the circulatory vessel. The thrombus can damage the valves of the vein and its lining. Some examples are physical injury like getting hit with a baseball bat or fellow soccer player, previous DVT, veins removed for surgical harvests (veins used in heart surgery for bypass), catheters, burns, and getting kicked every night in the calf by a significant other when trying to sleep since she or he has "Restless Leg Syndrome."

2) Stasis is basically sluggish flow. Sitting or standing for a long time without movement, obesity, sedentary life style, paralysis or paresis (weakness) from neurological disorders, congestive heart failure, pulmonary hypertension,

advancing age, anatomical variations in the circulatory system, and varicose veins. Liver and kidney disease as well as pregnancy which slows the flow and can produce a pro-thrombotic state (a propensity to produce a clot) making it a dual threat. One wonders that if someone had "Restless Leg Syndrome" are they at less risk for a thrombosis due to the incessant movement?

3) Hypercoagulability is by far the most complex and this rubric possesses the most etiologies. It is embedded in that awful figure 1 where the coagulation cascade gets disturbed. The medicines that are used to treat venous thromboembolism affect those illustrated pathways albeit in different ways. It would be too numerous to list every possible disease but I will attempt to break them up into general categories with some examples.

Active cancer; recent surgeries; inflammatory diseases like Crohn's disease and ulcerative colitis; medicines including birth control pills; hormonal replacement-both male and female; pregnancy; infections like HIV and the swine flu; cirrhosis of the liver; autoimmune diseases like lupus; smoking; obesity; certain kidney disorders; and lastly and what I believe are the most inscrutable, the often genetically tucked away thrombophilia.

It is in my view that the latter poses the most hazard because they are silently loitering. Just about all the other causes are either obvious or are diagnosed prior to any thrombosis. Certainly the autoimmune diseases are not so apparent but today's healthcare providers are screening more for them. Rarely does a disease like HIV or ulcerative colitis present with a thrombus. A good history will allow the physician to know a patient's medicines and though Trousseau sign (a venous thrombosis associated with certain malignancies) is taught to every first year medical student, it is indeed rare. Unfortunately the finding usually portends a particularly bad prognosis where the patient unfortunately succumbs to the cancer not a pulmonary embolism. In fact the eponymous Armand Trousseau who first described the sign later found it on himself and soon died from pancreatic cancer. I guess one should be careful for which one becomes famous?

About 10% of cancer patients will develop a clinically diagnosed DVT which is a rate 6 times higher than those without cancer. It appears that not all cancers are created equally as brain cancer, multiple myeloma (bone), gastric cancer (stomach), and pancre- 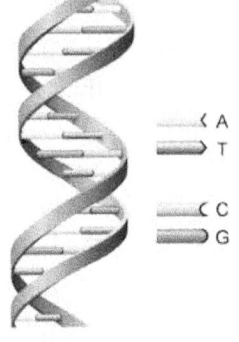 atic cancer have a higher potential for developing a hypercoagulable state. Lung cancer, lymphoma, and gynecologic cancers are not too far behind. The administration of chemotherapeutic drugs themselves can be extremely damaging to the blood vessels, making them susceptible to clotting.

FIGURE 2: DNA

So what are these mysterious inherited thrombophilia disorders arising from DNA mutations that produce either too much, too little, or dysfunctional clotting proteins? First that cameo appearance of science that I talked about in the introduction. Just a smidgeon about inheritance, DNA, and what a protein is.

DNA which stands for deoxyribonucleic acid is basically a twisted ladder made up of trillions of chemical bases. Each side of the ladder has a backbone of alternating sugars and phosphate (a chemical) groups. Attached to each sugar is one of four bases. The bases are adenine, thymine, guanine, and cytosine and are designated as A, T, G, and C. The two sides (strands) are held together by bonds between the bases. Each 3 letter code represents an amino acid. Currently we know of 22 natural amino acids (20 universal, 2 variant). The genetic code is the relation between the sequence of bases in DNA (or its RNA transcripts) and the sequence of amino acids in proteins.

Proteins consist of large molecules composed of one or more long chains of amino acids. An example of a DNA coding segment is ACG-CGG-ACG. If there is a spelling error then that represents a mutation which can cause a protein to change shape or make the body produce the wrong amount. The prothrombin gene mutation G20210A gets its name because an A (the base adenine) is substituted for a G (the base guanine) at the 20210st position of the protein's alphabet.

Thrombophilia is considered a dominant trait. This means that a person only has to have one mutation in one of his/her two gene copies to have the condition. If one copy is affected then they are said to be heterozygous. If both copies one from each parent, then the term homozygous is used. If they are homozygous then they are at greater risk for a clot then someone who is heterozygous. If one parent does not have the mutation and the other is homozygous then their offspring will have the mutation since the affected parent does not have a mutation free copy to pass on. If the affected parent is heterozygous then there is a 50:50 chance of transmission to the offspring as the good copy may be transmitted statistically half the time. Genetic counselors are available to interpret the possible permutations based on the genetics of both parents.

With that out of the way the following are the more commonly encountered congenital disorders with some accompanying information.

1) Factor V Leiden: This protein's production is controlled by other proteins including protein C and protein S which help break up the clot-producing factor V. This thrombophilia is a mutated form of factor V resisting inactivation. 1 out of 20 Caucasians have factor V Leiden. About 1% of African Americans, Hispanic Americans, and Native Americans have the mutation. It is rarely found in Asians. In people with a thrombosis 10% have this modification. The alteration was first identified in 1994 by researchers in Leiden (Netherlands).

2) Prothrombin gene mutation G20210A: The change in the prothrombin gene is present in 2-4% of Caucasians and .4% of African Americans. People with this variation make too much prothrombin. It is found in 5-10% of people with a thrombosis. Remember we named the factors? This is factor II in the aforementioned mnemonic: Foolish **People (prothrombin)**............

3) Protein C and S deficiencies: .2% of the general population have this deficiency. It is found in 2.5-6% of people with thrombosis. The prevalence of protein S deficiency in the general population is not known but it is found in 1.3-5% of patients with a thrombosis. Protein C deficiency can cause a severe clotting disorder in the newborn as well as the adult. Protein C and S deficiencies has been associated with necrosis of the skin upon starting a patient on blood thinner.

4) Resistance to activated Protein C: If this is found then there is a 95% chance that the person has a mutation of the factor V gene.

5) Plasminogen and plasminogen activator abnormalities: Tissue plasminogen activator (tPA) is an enzyme that helps dissolve clots. It is produced in the cells lining the blood vessels but if not functioning properly or there is not enough, clotting can become exaggerated. tPA is used in clinical medicine as a thrombolytic (clot buster).

6) Fibrinogen abnormalities- factor I: During normal coagulation a protein called thrombin converts fibrinogen to fibrin strands which help make up a clot. Too much fibrinogen and clotting can be exuberant. Smoking and inflammation can increase fibrinogen levels. The message is clear don't smoke.

7) Antithrombin deficiency: The term antithrombin was coined in 1905 describing the plasma's (colorless part of the blood) ability to neutralize thrombin which is part of the clotting cascade. It is primarily synthesized in the liver. If the liver is not functioning properly then less is

produced and that deficiency can lead to a potential clot. This is one of the reasons why people with cirrhosis have a propensity for VTE. .2% of the general population has this congenital deficiency. It is found in .5-.75% of those with a thrombosis.

8) Elevated levels of factors VIII and IX: These factors along with factor V are activated when thrombin is generated. People who have type O blood have a ¼ to ½ risk of having a thrombosis compared to those with other blood groups because there are reduced levels of factor VIII.

9) Factor XIII mutation: A deficiency of this factor is rare but can cause life-threatening hemorrhage. Bizarrely alterations in its levels predisposes one to thrombosis.

Some prevalence data is not known due to its relative scarcity. The most common are factor V Leiden and the prothrombin G20210A mutation. They are generally considered mild in relation to the other disorders.

There are also acquired thrombophilia such as the antiphospholipid syndrome which can also produce an arterial thrombosis and cause issues in pregnant women as do some of the inherited disorders. In the antiphospholipid syndrome there are antibodies that attack the cell membrane. This was first recognized in lupus patients and is associated with migraine headaches. If a woman has as a history of miscarriages, stillbirths, or complicated pregnancies her obstetrician will check for these disorders.

Heparin induced thrombocytopenia (low platelets) abbreviated as HIT, and paroxysmal nocturnal hemoglobinuria abbreviated as PNH can cause abnormal clotting. Indeed it is a bit cryptic but both blood thinners heparin and warfarin can cause clotting via complex biochemical reactions under specific conditions. Sickle cell disease and certain myloproliferative disorders where too many cells are mass produced by the bone marrow can also lead to thrombosis. There appears to be an association with the protein homocysteine which has been implicated in atherosclerosis (hardening and narrowing of the arteries), heart attacks, strokes, and possibly Alzheimer's disease.

Although not entirely understood elevated levels of factors I, VIII, IX, XI, XIII are associated with venous thrombosis.

These groups of both genetic and acquired diseases are out there in the medical periphery and are by no means in the forefront of the primary care physician's cerebrum no matter how astute. They have their hands full with just diabetes, hypertension, and elevated cholesterol while wrestling with the nascent health care system.

Testing for these disorders is expensive and in a paradigm where the words "healthcare and cost cutting" are enjoined, mass screening does not appear to be on the horizon. Nor should it.

Since 1977 I have read every year a book entitled "Current Medical Diagnosis and Treatment. (CMDT)." The biggest change from CMDT 1977 through CMDT 2016 is that there is more and more information, more and more available tests, and almost an unbelievable amount of genetic testing options.

Just recently Angelina Jolie's preventive bilateral mastectomy had been performed after assessment of her family history along with a BRCA1 and BRCA2 gene analysis. Inherited mutations in these genes increase the risk for female breast and ovarian cancers. To my knowledge these tests run around $3000. Not a problem for Mrs. Brad Pitt but the pendulum (I couldn't resist) speaks to the many ethical issues. Healthcare insurance companies and governments need to watch their bottom line. They cannot nor should they be expected to pay for every available test known to man. But in my view there are situations where these tests should be (later). But which ones and what situations? Who determines which tests and what situations? The government, the insurance company, a specialist, the patient, a panel of doctors and ethicists? How about the United States Congress but only when their approval rating climbs to double-digits. Don't hold your breath.

That being addressed the United States in my humble opinion does not need to have every new technological weapon multiplied by a factor of 100 in case of World War 13. This speaks to America's allocation of financial resources.

So ostensibly the duel between Otto Bismarck and Dr. Rudolf Virchow really was not cancelled. It continues worldwide over a century later and my guess for centuries to follow.

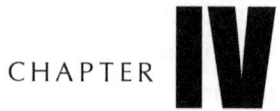

SIGNS & SYMPTOMS of WHAT FEELS LIKE the END TIMES

NOW THAT WE have some understanding of VTE how do we recognize its presence in real time? First let us differentiate between a sign and a symptom.

A symptom is what the patient experiences and is generally subjective. A sign is what anybody recognizes and is objective. The patient shows up with the symptom of an "ear ache," the provider looks inside the ear canal with an otoscope and sees a red tympanic membrane (eardrum). The symptom is the ache, the sign is the redness. The physician cannot feel the patient's ache nor can the patient look into his or her ear. Even if it were possible the patient may not apprehend that there is an abnormality as they have had no visual experience of what a normal eardrum looks like. Now they are not always deracinated. A patient can emerge complaining of a symptomatic rash and the physician literally sees it as a sign of trouble. The 2 terms are often confused as it theoretically depends as to whom is doing the observing. With that confusion made worse what are the symptoms and signs of a VTE? Well as mentioned before there may be none. Autopsies have been performed that reveal pulmonary emboli that were silent. But when there are issues beheld what is the presentation? In the case of deep vein thrombosis one may experience calf swelling, have a leg ache like a Charlie horse or experience pain on walking. There may be a sensation of warmth to the affected leg, engorged surface veins, and leg fatigue. In the case of a pulmonary embolism there are symptoms like chest pain, shortness of breath (dyspnea), fast heart rate (tachycardia), fever(pyrexia), rapid breathing (tachypnea), and cough even with blood (hemoptysis), anxiety, and dizziness. The physician may observe changes in the heart sounds as well as rate and rhythm, neck vein distention, blue lips (cyanosis), blood pressure swings, swelling of the legs, hear fluid in your lungs (rales), and observe sweating.

The examiner will try to distinguish if it is a provoked PE which is determined if there are recent (3 months) transient major risk factors like surgery, hormone administration, or immobility vs. an unprovoked PE where there are no recent potentials but the patient has active cancer, a family history of VTE, or thrombophilia. The unprovoked is so named because the patient did not bring it on voluntarily.

In fact there are actual algorithmic tables attempting to collate signs and symptoms. One is the PERC (Pulmonary

Embolism Rule out Criteria), another The Revised Geneva Scoring System, and yet another The Wells Prediction Rule Well Criteria. Basically these are tables with numbers assigned to the signs and symptoms. They are added up and depending on the score the probability decided. There have been some articles in the medical literature positing that these charts are helpful but ultimately the gut feeling of an experienced physician is more dependable. "Kickin' It Old Skool" if you like stupid movies.

Whether by criteria or intuition a special X-ray called a CT-angiogram will be ordered if there is a suspicion of a PE. Of course now that every emergency room has access to CT-angiograms the frequency of this test being ordered is recently up over 10% during the last 15 years. Unfortunately the mortality from PE has barely budged during that same time period. Aside from the additional healthcare costs one wonders if we will see an increase in cancers from the extra ionized radiation given to patients with shortness of breath and chest discomfort. The diagnostics will be discussed in chapter 5. But for now the bottom line is this, if one is experiencing any of these manifestations one needs to leave this short chapter and go to the next one. That is the emergency room because there are many possibilities when dealing with this symptom complex. Some examples are panic attack, heart attack, pleurisy (inflammation of the lung's lining), gall bladder disease, gastrointestinal reflux (GERD), pneumonia, arthritis of the spine, torn esophagus (swallowing tube),aneurysm (ballooning of an artery), pericarditis(inflammation of heart lining), shingles, asthma, bronchitis, pneumothorax (lung collapse), or something as harmless as inflamed muscles around the rib cage.

Chest pain in itself is a very common presentation and emergency rooms have chest pain monitoring protocols to separate the wheat from the chaff so to speak. Some hospitals even have chest pain centers.

The important thing to remember is that chest pain deserves a sober inquiry and must be professionally evaluated. Even if one is pretty sure as to what is causing the discomfort, one needs to get tests to rule out the possible etiologies. It is too easy to be indisputably dead wrong. A person needs to be wrong only once and it could be the last decision they ever make.

CHAPTER V

LAMENTATIONS
THE EMERGENCY ROOM &
BEYOND

WHEN ONE DRIVES by their neighborhood sick bays on a Saturday night on the way to dinner the eyes may catch the glimpse of the neon EMERGENCY ROOM sign often in red and one thinks nothing of it. When short of breath and feeling that death is near, it means everything.

Depending on the symptoms one may have very well driven oneself or was taken in an emergency vehicle, sirens and all. There are a few ways that pulmonary embolisms will present- no warning (where you would continue driving to dinner), mild-moderate symptomatic, severely symptomatic, and do I have a living will symptomatic?

Let us assume for now that the patient is a 55 year old Afro-American female with moderate symptoms and that she drove herself to a hospital or urgent care center. The regimen for the other presentations will briefly be addressed later.

She came in breathless and anxious and relayed to the front desk that she was having chest pain and could not breathe. She will be immediately taken to triage usually by a nurse. Her birthday, name, and date are put on a wrist band and applied. A rapid history is taken as electrocardiogram (EKG) leads are placed on her chest and someone notifies the doc that there is a patient with chest pain. The EKG is unremarkable and she is taken to an uncomfortable bed in the emergency department. There she will be given a gown while someone places an IV (intravenous) line in her arm and draws a formatted chest pain lab panel. She is asked "What brought you in tonight?" More history- hers' and her family history is taken and typed into the computer." Height and weight?" "What medicines are you on? ""Do you smoke or drink or use any illicit drugs?" "Previous surgeries and any other medical problems?" "Who is your doctor?" The good people are trying to keep her calm as she is wired up to some amazing technology. Blood pressure, pulse, heart rate, and blood oxygen levels are constantly being recorded. A cursory physical is done with attention to lung sounds via a stethoscope and a glance at the lower extremities with a squeeze or two. The physician, probably a resident (doctor in training) may try to elicit Homan's sign which is when the knee is fully extended the foot is forcibly dorsiflexed (pushed towards the head) to see if it produces any pain. Recently this maneuver has fallen out of favor as the procedure itself can dislodge a deep vein thrombosis and send it to the lung. In the practice of medicine and in most other human endeavors the only thing that stays the same is change.

Fortunately her vital signs are stable and she is given some extra oxygen nasally. After a few nurses, maybe a physician assistant, and someone to recheck address, insurance, birthday, etc. the attending physician appears and digs a bit deeper as to why she is in "his" or "her" emergency department on Saturday night. The "his "or "her" may be verbally accentuated depending on the amount of REM sleep and coffee the emergency room doctor has had. The physician will also do an examination. The only thing of note is that she has some mild hypertension which runs in the family along with diabetes and that she is on hormone replacement therapy (HRT) for menopause. As this is going on the labs are being run.

The differential diagnosis for chest pain as previously mentioned is quite vast so the interrogation will be more targeted. "Have you ever had anxiety, gall bladder disease, ulcers, spine or rib issues, recent fevers, heartburn, swallowing issues, rashes, stomach pain, cough, snoring, nausea, vomiting, dizziness?" Describe the chest pain-sharp, squeezing, vise-like?" The physician's brain is running human algorithms to ascertain what is most likely. The labs returned and everything looked pretty good except a test called the D-Dimer. It is 3x normal. At that moment the data processing stops at the most likely diagnosis of VTE.

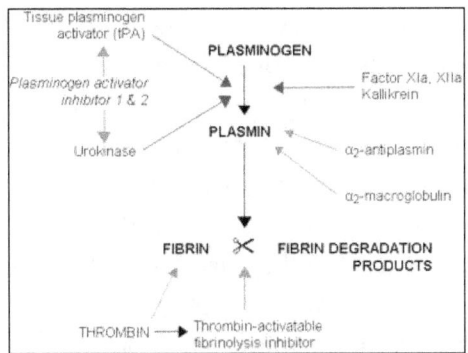

FIGURE 3: CLOT DISSOLUTION.

The D-Dimer is basically a fibrin degradation product (shown above) of a process called fibrinolysis that dissolves clots. If the D-Dimer is 3x normal rest assure that there is at least one thrombus and your body is already on the job. The D-Dimer test has revolutionized the diagnosis of VTE but like all things in medicine it is not perfect. The test results can be equivocal as a person's age has some effect on the cut-offs of what is normal versus abnormal. There is a possibility in the future that age-adjusted D-Dimer assays may be what is ordered.

The future is now however, so our patient is whisked away to the X-ray department where an ultrasound to scan her lower extremities will be done. Sometimes impedance plethysmography is performed which is a test that measures changes in electrical impedance along the vessel. However most emergency room evaluations involve Doppler technology. Ironically the reference standard for the diagnosis of DVT called contrast venography, where dye is injected into the vein to look for a filling defect has also lost most of its previous shine. Then off to another section of the radiology department to get a chest X-ray basically to rule out other entities and the all-important CTA (CAT scan angiogram) of your chest. The CTA is a CAT scan administered with contrast material so the radiologist can get a good look at the arteries at different levels. It is a great diagnostic test but there is about a 15-20% false negative rate, meaning that your clot(s) are missed. Thankfully it appears that those escaping detection are often clinically insignificant. The safe but invasive pulmonary angiogram where dye is injected to visualize the arteries is the gold standard for PE diagnosis but its appropriate role in most cases is debatable.

When I was a physician in training the ventilation-perfusion lung scan (VQ scan) was popular where radio-labeled albumin (a protein) was injected into a vein and allowed to travel to the pulmonary circulation. Then the patient would breathe a gas or aerosol while the radioactivity in the lungs was recorded. A perfusion defect represented decreased flow to the region. Unfortunately many findings were not specific and we had to decoct the reports based on probabilities. Despite the imperfect CTA, it is infinitely better as compared to the VQ scan. Since the arrival at the emergency ward was at night these images will probably be sent to the radiologist on call via the institution's Intranet where they can be viewed on a personal computer.

Imagine a life hanging in the balance and waiting for somebody who may very well be in a bathrobe viewing computer porn to make the diagnosis. You Have Mail!!!!!!!!!!!! 70% of the time that there is pulmonary embolism a DVT will be detected by the concomitant ultrasound. In our patient's case she was found to be in the majority when "Long John Radiologist" sent the reports to the emergency room via the same secured connection.

Thrombolysis (the bursting of clots) may restore patency in the occluded leg veins and decrease the post thrombotic syndrome but it does not decrease your chances of having a PE. Additionally thrombolysis is associated with more bleeding complications and does nothing to decrease mortality. There is some data suggesting that by threading a catheter directly to the thrombus and injecting the "clot buster" that results are better but more head to head studies are required. It is recommended that in cases of impending venous gangrene that thrombolysis be used. I bring this up because in the practice of medicine rarely are things either black or white. Gangrene is most definitely black.

The currently "approved" treatment options are basically three and these are simplified for the reader. The 1st option involves hospitalization for about 2- 5 days starting IV unfractionated (not important) heparin and oral warfarin known to many by the moniker Coumadin. Both as previously mentioned are blood thinners. The heparin prevents further thrombi until the warfarin starts to work as measured by a laboratory test called an INR (International Normalized Ratio). Warfarin, an acronym for the Wisconsin Alumni Research Foundation is about 60 years old and is the main ingredient in rat poison. It is important to note that neither drug breaks up clots, it prevents new ones while your body does the work through fibrinolysis (Figure 2). This is an expensive regime because of the prolonged hospitalization and is being supplanted by option two.

Option 2 is low molecular weight (also not important) heparin or a drug named Arixtra (fondaparinux) given sub-cutaneously (an injection under the skin). A prescription for warfarin will be given prior to leaving the ward that day, no hospitalization. Outpatient treatment for PE is not universally accepted but the Canadians seem to be more comfortable with it. I personally think it will be the standard of care everywhere. An INR will get checked as an outpatient in 2-3 days. Either option will entail stopping the heparin when the INR is considered therapeutic which is in the 2-3 range. Some physicians like the range 2-3.5. Normal is 1. Warfarin will be continued for a period of time based on if the VTE was determined as provoked or not provoked. It will in all probability be assumed it was the former based on the estrogen use but that might only be one factor. Three to six months of treatment should be anticipated.

Once the INRs are deemed stable the seemingly incessant visits to the laboratory can be reduced. Coumadin is a vitamin K antagonist (VKA) and inhibits the synthesis of the coagulation factors II, VII, IX, and X which depend on the vitamin. Ironically the drug initially inhibits proteins C and S which are natural anticoagulants. Sometimes there is a coagulation factor imbalance that leads to a paradoxical hypercoagulable state and thrombosis.

A diet sheet will be given explaining what foods are high in vitamin K, mostly green leafy vegetables. Kale is loaded with vitamin K along with calcium and should be best avoided in larger quantities. One does not need stop these foods but keep them moderately consistent on a quotidian basis. Coumadin is a tricky drug. Even a moderate extra serving of kale can drop an INR below 2 and thus expose one to more thrombosis formation. If the INR gets too high the risk of hemorrhage increases. Quite frankly the endless monitoring can make one crazy.

Advice regarding gradient stockings to wear so post thrombotic syndrome (PTS) can hopefully be obviated will be discussed. The problem it seems that though these special stockings can diminish leg edema (swelling) and pain, recent studies have shown that they do not prevent fully the complication which can affect 40% of those who had a DVT. Like I said the "practice" of medicine.

Good news for the patient is that she survived the 1st critical hours of a moderate VTE and will be out of the hospital soon. But is she out of the woods? Not necessarily.

The next chapter we discuss the possible aftermath of this major bodily insult. But first let us discuss treatment option 3 and the two other possible presentations that gives one an inkling to go to the hospital and not supper- the severely symptomatic and the about- to- die brand.

Option 3 involves a new class of drugs called the Xa inhibitors used in place of warfarin. On television one might have seen commercials for Pradaxa (dabigatran),

Xarelto (rivaroxaban), and Eliquis (apixaban) regarding the treatment of atrial fibrillation (abnormal heart rhythm). Basically this burgeoning drug class does not treat the arrhythmia but helps prevent clots and strokes associated with the cardiac irregularity. So far advertising for the Xa inhibitors and its role in VTE has been scant. Even Madison Avenue appears to be treating embolic disease as purely secondary which helps keep the general public blissfully ignorant. A recent study called the Einstein Study (not Virchow) showed these drugs to be non-inferior to heparin and Coumadin. I am not sure Albert would have liked the hyphenated conclusion.

There is no INR monitoring, no bridging with heparin, and no dietary restrictions. There is however no easy way to reverse the Xa inhibitor effects upon mistakenly taking a handful thinking they were M and M candies. The FDA did just recently approved a drug called Praxbind (idarucizumab) to reverse the anticoagulant actions of Pradaxa. I imagine other reversal drugs are in the pipeline. They are very expensive but my guess is that the Xa inhibitors will be included into the standard of care regimen when less expensive generics as well as antidotes are available. Most warfarin can then be saved primarily for the rats. Hopefully the rodents don't find kale chips while hunting for cheese as that would make warfarin *less -superior*. Ugh!

If one was to arrive with a PE and was unstable the doctor would use the drugs mentioned above for dissolving the DVT called thrombolytics. This time since the monster has already traveled to the lung. Despite the possibility of a bleeding complication this treatment is not questionable requiring more studies. The attending physician would not want to wait for the body's own fibrinolysis (diagram above) because the vital signs are poor and if the thrombus is not lysed soon the chance of death increases. The majority of studies are indicating that thrombolysis be used only for the large embolisms. There are those that feel the drug class could be administered for the sub-large group depending on other factors. The current data suggests that thrombolytic therapy hastens clot resolution during the first 24 hours but at 1 week and 1 month there is no difference in outcomes when compared to heparin and warfarin.

If one arrived to the hospital in extremis he or she would be rushed to surgery, after a stat pulmonary angiogram, (dye directly placed in your arterial system) and an attempt to extract the embolus surgically once the test shows where the embolism is. This is called an embolectomy and reserved for those near death. These are the massive embolisms often with huge clot burdens in key arterial branches. It does not get much worse than this from a prognostic standpoint.

Interestingly in 2014 a European study demonstrated that the location of the coagulum is more important than the burden of the clot in most patients. An embolus that takes up residence in the central part of the lung even if the patient is hemodynamically stable, appears to generate more mischief than its peripheral neighbors. Homeowner associations beware!

So just to summarize on the subject of treatment, it initially begins with the patient recognizing that something just is not right, then an emergency evaluation followed by a judicious choice from a panoply of pharmaceutical drugs. Possibly accompanying the choices are IVC filters (next chapter), anti-embolism stockings, and surgical intervention if required.

What hasn't been discussed thus far regarding treatment is belief that you will get better. In order to recover from this devastating disease one must have conviction that you will. A subject so complex, ideational, and controversial that it will have a dedicated chapter in Medusa's Clot.

Who is this chick Medusa one might be wondering at this point? She in Greek mythology was the rather unfortunate looking snake-haired termagant whose face if directly gazed upon turned the unsuspecting viewer into a stone-hard corpse as their breath was slowly taken from them. The wench was eventually decapitated by the hero Perseus as he viewed her indirectly through the reflection of his polished shield.

I am afraid a sword just won't cut it if we have any chance of eradicating the wretched brute of pulmonary embolism.

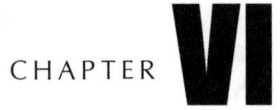

AFTERMATH: PHYSICIAN HEAL THYSELF?

THERE ARE THOSE who after experiencing VTE are up and about relatively quickly. Others have complications ranging from fatigue, hemoptysis (coughing up blood), palpitations, heart failure, pulmonary hypertension, chronic dyspnea (shortness of breath) to shock and sudden death. Much is dependent on as those selling real estate like to say "location-location!" In another words where did the embolism ultimately wind up taking up residence. Other factors are age, general health, mental attitude and other co-morbidities. Quite frankly I think much is luck intertwined with your personal genome.

Many including myself have a ghastly course. There are VTE discussion groups on the Internet that are quite enlightening as their sequelae is discussed in length. Many are suffering from continual chest pain, shortness

of breath, anxiety, depression, and just plain old unadulterated fear. This is not an easy way to wade through life.
What is particularly disturbing is that rarely on discharge
from the hospital are these symptoms discussed orally or
in written form. Moreover many of these manifestations
are identical to the symptoms that made the patient go the
emergency room in the first place.

Numerous patients have returned to the emergency
rooms and had all their tests repeated and most showed
some clot resolution given some time. Some showed more
clot burden. Other people it was discovered also had a
blockage of their heart arteries and needed coronary intervention. One person posted that he had showers of
more emboli despite having a "good" INR (International
Normalized Ratio) and needed a filter placed in the big
vein called the inferior vena cava to hopefully catch the
rest.

These filters were a bit more popular in the past. There
are issues of increased post-phlebitic syndrome after inser-
tion and the strainer itself can dislodge essentially making
itself a foreign body embolism. There are instances that
IVC (inferior vena cava) interruption is absolutely recommended. Those who cannot tolerate anticoagulation and
patients who have recurrent embolisms despite adequate
anticoagulation (patient in the above discussion group).
Consideration is given to patients with unstable INR levels and who are non-compliant with their blood thinners.
Additionally bariatric patients, with a BMI (body mass index) greater than 55 undergoing surgery for weight control

and having other risk factors may be candidates.

The filters are usually inserted using an ultrasound guided micro-puncture or needle into the jugular (neck) or femoral (leg) vein with fluoroscopy (continuous X-ray image) and threaded to the IVC. The procedure is usually performed by an interventional radiologist or vascular surgeon. These products come in two flavors, retrievable and non-retrievable. The temporary umbrella-like filters, when indicated are inserted for a short inter-critical period.

These post insult symptoms are not easily explainable in today's medical paradigm and have not found a comfortable home in the accessible vernacular. Most healthcare providers think this is a psychological overreaction and to a degree they are right but not for a lack of reason. I am convinced that if they experienced a PE they would not throw that term around in such a loose fashion. There is bruited about the term "Post Pulmonary Embolism Syndrome" which describes the symptoms. Numerous explanations from continued pleurisy (inflammation of the lung's lining), remodeling of arteries, and neurologically (via nerves) mediated reflexes to the psychiatric responses to it.

It is interesting that when one has a heart attack (myocardial infarction) there is often a prescribed rehabilitation sequence. There are cardiac centers who just specialize in getting patients back on their feet but after a pulmonary embolism there really is nothing despite the draconian psychological and physical deconditioning that it often produces. Sometimes a pulmonary embolism is associated with a pulmonary infarction where lung tissue is killed.

After a provoked or unprovoked VTE one needs to make changes. Alterations in the medical regimen may be required as well as life style changes. Tobacco is taboo and if obese one needs to lose weight. Also if one has a sedentary existence one needs to make it less so. These changes are often difficult but it is imperative to reduce the chances of having another event because there is a higher fortuity because of the previous PE. Simple tasks like taking a trip for more than 2 hours will now require getting up and about or wiggling your legs to keep the claret liquid flowing. The use of gradient stockings to promote good flow in the legs are often difficult to work with especially if one is a male. Not to mention future medical visits, possible diagnostic work ups, needle sticks if on Coumadin, and those wonderful pill boxes at bedside. One week I had four different appointments. I was so tired of filling out the same premonitory questionnaire that when it came to the questions about marriage and sex I answered "occasionally" & less occasionally." The receptionist was bemused.

Watching the types of foods one eats regarding vitamin K (Coumadin loses its effectiveness with increased vitamin K) and being on the lookout for excess bleeding of the gums, bruising, and blood in the stools, urine, and sputum. Certain medicines for a simple headache like Advil are to be avoided when on blood thinners. Those women still menstruating may see higher or longer flows and can easily become anemic. Shaving can be an adventure. When lab studies are drawn the nurse or technician will keep pressure on the puncture site longer.

There is a whole set of criteria regarding blood thinners and dental work, joint injections, minor and major surgeries, as well as other medical procedures. These molecules are very labor intensive especially if they are prescribed for the rest of your life.

This Post PE Syndrome can last for months and some still experience issues years later. Lost wages, gradual deconditioning, increased fatigue, and hopelessness coupled with interpersonal conflicts can put a lot of stress on any loving relationship. Like a nuclear armament detonated, the effects goes on long afterwards.

I drove myself to the emergency room in 2013 after experiencing mild chest discomfort and politely said at the desk that I had chest pain and had a history of pulmonary embolism. The routine from the last chapter went into motion. All the preliminary studies but one came back and were rather pristine as were my vital signs. The nurse implied that I was over reacting, or at least that is what I inferred. I nicely asked her if the D-Dimer was back and if it was not would she be interested in making a wager that it was abnormal. She demurred at the suggestion. When the study did eventually turn up it was at an egregious level of 3500, approximately 7x higher than normal. I think she said that was a record. A Pyrrhic victory I would have preferred not on my resume. Great maybe the hospital will name a wing after me. Ugh!

I was admitted and discharged the next day with the bare minimum "routine" discharge directions. The chest pains and breathing got worse as I was running back and forth to the laboratory on a near daily basis getting my INR checked. In the morning I would give myself a subcutaneous injection of Lovenox, a heparin formulation we had touched upon. During the first week I was lucky to get in touch with one of my old intern buddies who was a superb general internist and he was kind enough to take care of me. Within 3 days of my discharge I could not sit up without profound dyspnea (shortness of breath). The condition is opposite of those who are in heart failure who cannot lie down without getting short of breath because the blood return to the diseased heart is rapid and furious in that position. What I was experiencing was called platypnea (shortness of breath while sitting up) which usually indicates some kind of blood shunting (abnormal pathway) within the circulatory system or liver involvement. I used to quiz my medical students about the weird symptom, one that I never heard a patient complain about.

I was convinced that I was in big trouble and was referred to a heart specialist and hematologist to rule out any genetic diseases. Both physicians were coevals and both tried to assuage my fears. Unfortunately they could not and in the interim one of the genetic tests came back positive for the prothrombin gene mutation, simply abbreviated as G20210A. Prothrombin is factor II in the coagulation cascade and is the second most common thrombophilia gene mutation in the population. I always knew my parents screwed me up emotionally but not genetically? To make things worse I was trying to keep my children from learning about my hospitalization and illness as not to worry them. Now I had to let all my first degree relatives know so they should be tested. I was particularly concerned about my daughter as she was on pro-thrombotic medicines in the past and might one day be on them again or become pregnant. Both are risk factors for VTE.

I was more concerned for my two children as I was for myself. I was convinced that I was in a bad subset of those who suffered a PE. Some complications are extremely frightening so if one does not mind a little redundancy: right heart infarction and failure, chronic embolic showers, and chronic pulmonary hypertension (increase blood pressure of the lung arteries). I just wanted my kids to be okay. My daughter tested fine. My son as usual rarely gets alarmed and will have the tests done at his next check-up. Probably 2030.

As time went on I pleaded with the internist to reorder the CAT scan but he felt I had enough radiation. I could not disagree with that possibility given all the procedures I had but my imagination was taking me into a bad place especially when sitting up. The dyspnea also worsened with coffee ingestion. I just kept imagining that this rather large bloody concoction was sending its little particulate scions deeper into my arteries. My friend referred me to a psychiatrist as he felt I was losing it. Quite frankly I agreed with him. The cardiologist I had seen did an echocardiogram (ultrasound of the heart) which was essentially within normal limits. My physical exam was within normal limits as were my vital signs. The psychiatrist thought I was suffering from post-traumatic stress disorder, depression, and anxiety. Some anti-depressant medicine was prescribed but I of course had an adverse reaction to it. My wheels were beginning to feel very wobbly. To complicate matters prior to my VTE I was on topical testosterone due to a bilateral orchiectomy (testicles were removed). Hormone replacement is associated not only with heart disease but with thrombus formation so I went off the drug which produced mood disorder issues and "Seinfeld-shrinkage" of the one remaining genitalia I had left. I also was wearing gradient stockings up to my knees. Could tampons be far off as well as a name change from Michael to Michelle Caitlin?

Needless to say things were not going very well and on Black Friday, the day after Thanksgiving, I was rushed back to the emergency room with labored breathing and chest pain via an ambulance. I was asking G-d for help at about the 5 mile mark. A repeat ultrasound of the legs and CAT scan of the chest showed near resolution of the clot. I began to breathe easier with the results which was at the three week anniversary. You really can worry yourself to death.

I wish I could say that I felt great and it was all in my head which I was beginning to think. The month of December was better but I would still out of the blue get chest pain and labored breathing but it was tolerable. I was able to sit up more and for longer periods. That came in handy because it was easier to reread on the Internet the 4.9 million web pages on pulmonary embolism. I was told it would take time, that I had a major insult to a major organ, and just wait it out. I think the major organ was my brain.

I did wait it out until my favorite weekend of the NFL, the Wild Card games and everything crashed including my Philadelphia Eagles who lost by a field goal to the New Orleans Saints. I never saw the game because I was back at the hospital emergency room and to make matters more absurd the television was not working. All the tests were repeated and the record setting D- Dimer was now a normal 200 as were the repeat ultrasound and CAT scans.

I was admitted that night to Abington Hospital for cardiac monitoring as everyone appeared stumped. I saw another cardiologist in the morning who thought it was safe for me to go home but he ordered a repeat echocardiogram and stress test to evaluate my possible broken heart. The tests were done the following week and were normal. With that information I felt better and with his great bedside manner he tried to convince me that though I had an atypical presentation I would ultimately be fine. His optimism, though appreciated still seemed off the mark because the symptoms were not typical given the time passed.

He thought that it was a combination of post-traumatic stress, generalized anxiety, and physiological changes still going on at the pulmonary level. He also said I was terrifyingly bright (he evidently was not quite awake) and that made things worse. I remember that early Sunday morning conversation almost verbatim. I replied that I was anything but bright but in my desire to care properly for my patients I made myself ill. He looked at me whimsically. I explained that at the end of the day I found myself knowing less and less about more and more. My father once warned me as a little boy "Don't let the sun set on your ignorance." I soon realized like many of his other aphorisms the impossibility of heeding that admonition. Danielle Ofri of slate.com calls it "The Tyranny of Perfection." The practice of medicine is a harsh mistress. As a voracious autodidact who wanted to be familiar with nature "from from G-d down to the stones," I found myself frustrated. Now that I was the patient it was far more difficult and frightening. I explained to the heart specialist that I once saw a therapist who was attempting to show me the error in my driven ways. I almost did until she came down with an illness that her doctors could not figure out and she called me at some ungodly hour. After guiding her to the correct diagnosis I cancelled my further sessions. He laughed. Do as I say, not as I do. How about a rebate?

Nearly 10 years after "officially" retiring I still get up early every morning and listen to online medical lectures and read my favorite medical textbook for about an hour. Call me a bit compulsive but when one is sick, one wants a doctor who is not blissfully content with what he or she does not know. The good cardiologist understood because quite frankly it was evident to me that he was cut from the same cloth. It was 6am on a weekend after all. That sun my father spoke about was yet to rise that day on either of us. Tyranny indeed comes in many forms.

In essence what I indeed had was the abstruse Post Pulmonary Embolism Syndrome, a diagnosis for which I was lobbying others to make but they were unaware of the packaging. Two years after my pulmonary embolism I still get episodes of air hunger and chest discomfort, but they are not as frequent. At least I know what it is and what it is not. Certainly during times of stress or excess caffeine intake the symptoms appear more marked. Interestingly walking outside helps.

To this day I am unsure if this was a provoked or unprovoked pulmonary embolism or the often stated "combination of things." I certainly was sitting for a long time relatively dehydrated for hours at the casino and was on hormone replacement (provoked). I also have a thrombophilia (unprovoked). My first pulmonary embolism in 2006 was due to extreme listlessness after major lumbar spine surgery (provoked) but one wonders if and how much did the gene mutation contribute (unprovoked)? I was not on testosterone either back then.

For now I restarted the testosterone at 1/2 the dose, continue my lifetime blood thinners and hold my breath. It is absolutely frightening as it is mind-boggling. "Why me G-d? ""Why not fool?"

Prior to the 2013 PE I had an orthopedist, a physical therapist, a dentist, an audiologist and an urologist. Now I have in addition a cardiologist, a pulmonologist, an endocrinologist, a hematologist, a psychiatrist, a dermatologist (melanoma), and a general internist. What I really need is a hypnotist to get me to forget this stuff! I never wear jewelry but now wear a bracelet that says "Blood Thinners." I am still unsure if I should have the words facing towards me or away. Sartorially challenged to the end.

Go to stoptheclot.org or clotcare.com and one can read as many patient stories to a lung's content. Many people who posted had loved ones succumb to this killer. It is heart breaking.

Since we talked about Angelina Jolie and her impact on breast cancer awareness I have decided to include two celebrity chapters illustrating the two extremes of the co-agulation cascade, which is the source of all this nastiness. One is a problem with too much clotting, the other is one with not enough. You may wonder why discuss the latter? I have always been entrenched in the belief that if one wants to get a good grip on a subject then the two extremes should be understood. I can assure you for example that every offensive lineman playing football not only hones his skills at his position but also has a deep understanding of the defensive lineman's agenda. I think this goes for just about every other human endeavor. If one wants to be a better physician, become a patient and the perspective is forever enlightened. I would venture to say that there is not a good police officer out there who does not intimately understand the criminal faculty and is all the better for it. Is there any surprise that governments hire previous criminals to catch the current ones? Well I guess the point is made.

Prior to my sequential trips to Abington Hospital I had written an article in the paper about a horrible experience I had undergoing thyroid biopsies there about a month prior. I was not kind. Needless to say I owed it to the institution to write another missive from a different perspective. I was breathing a bit better so I was able to eat my crow sandwich and type. The following appeared in the Glenside News Globe Times.

LETTER: Return to Abington Hospital Shows Different Side of Institution

Published: Sunday, December 08, 2013

To the Editor:

In October, I wrote in this paper an excoriating letter about the draconian medical policies of the Abington Hospital Radiology Department. I went public because I did not get any response from the hospital's CEO after apprising him of the situation. Only after the missive was published did I receive a phone call from the hospital's Chief of Staff, Jack Kelly. He was gracious and apologetic, and he promised to remedy the situation. There was a part of me that wondered why it took the power of the press to generate a response? Was this just another overpaid bureaucrat doing some patronizing damage control? But when Kelly gave me his personal cell phone number I was persuaded to think that this was a good man doing a good job for a good hospital.

On Nov. 2, I suffered life-threatening pulmonary embolisms (clot). I was treated and released Nov. 3. Unfortunately, the symptoms of breathlessness, chest pain, and rapid heartbeat increased. Despite being reassured by multiple specialists that all would be well, things came to a crescendo on Black Friday and I was rushed to Abington

Hospital's first-class trauma center. I was just hoping that my "Most Wanted" picture wasn't hanging in the emergency room after torching the hospital's reputation.

I explained my situation to the most sentient staff. As we were awaiting the results of further tests, I called Kelly. He got right back to me and told me not to worry. The repeat CAT scan showed that the embolisms were almost gone, and with that information, the clinical complexion changed.

I humbly write this article because life is primarily written in a bimodal narrative, and by simply exposing the "bad" and not the "good" would make me infinitely and palpably worse. Is Abington Hospital 100 percent safe? Of course not. What hospital is?

Is Abington Hospital worth seeing? Yes, but like all hospitals, it isn't worth going to see it. There may be some truth to the outlandish Thomas Jefferson quote that "When doctors consult, vultures circle above," but those of us who have access to this less than perfect institution are lucky.

As for the actions of the lettered/physician bureaucrat Dr. J, he took my breath away and then helped give it back.

Dr. Michael Helzner

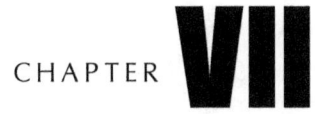

CHRONICLES (1)
DAVID BLOOM

LONG BEFORE REPORTER David Bloom went to Iraq to cover the war I was already a huge fan in the mid-1990s when he was NBC's White House correspondent. He appeared to have that inherent happy talent of elucidating communication and never feared to follow truth's timeline. He eventually became the anchor on Weekend Today which he hosted with Soledad O'Brien. He was a rising star with great television appeal along with cogent reporting. I thought one day he would be hosting the much sought after Nightly News. He eventually was assigned to cover the Middle East conflict in 2003. I remember watching this handsome guy in what was called the "Bloom Mobile" reporting on the battles and situations of the day. He was dressed as a soldier and appeared soldered to the floor of flatbed truck surrounded by an unbelievable amount of antennae.

Since Operation Desert Storm I was amazed how war was brought to the television in real time. I often wondered how the average citizen during Antiquity would have reacted being able to experience firsthand a battle on foreign soil. Additionally with all this technology combined with my amateur zeal for history I often wondered what my reaction would be to see Alexander the Great, Hannibal, Napoleon, or Genghis Khan in action. The other side of me finds it all rather vulgar to see war as a form of entertainment but people don't change just the technology. Nevertheless night after night I watched Mr. Bloom in his eponymous vehicle report the news.

I remember quite vividly when across the ticker on MSNBC came the sobering news that journalist David Bloom was killed in Iraq. My first thought was that he and members of the U.S. Third Infantry Division were killed by either bullets or explosives. I pictured him and his military companions bleeding to death in the middle of a barren sand heap. I could not have been more wrong. Mr. Bloom did not bleed to death, he essentially was coagulated to death. Mauled to death by a surreptitious clot(s).

As reports started filtering in and facts gathered it became known that he died from a pulmonary embolism. David Bloom collapsed under the Babylonian skies like so many warriors before him, and so many yet to follow. A young man not yet 40 killed in the middle of an American military operation from a thrombus that started in his legs and traveled to his lungs. Aside from the fact that I was upset over his passing, the physician part of me pictured a man standing for hours in high heat and being thrown about a bit by the uneven terrain. This scenario was also coupled with flights back and forth between New York and the Middle East. I also pondered that with the venous stasis and trauma along with probable dehydration did he have a hypercoagulable state?

When all the data was out he indeed had a genetic thrombophilia. It was purportedly the Factor V Leiden mutation. According to the reports he was complaining of leg cramps for days and his condition was relayed to physicians who suspected a DVT. When advised to seek care he refused, grabbed some aspirin and did what he did best, reported.

I am unsure if Mr. Bloom knew of his genetic propensity and if he indeed knew would he have taken that assignment? Looking at his personal history, at least one that can be gleaned from a computer screen he was quite the driven and ambitious sort. Could the reporter have been able to reign in his passions if his medical history and ramifications were realized is sadly a mere theoretical question? All we have are remnants. The only person who could have answered that question died in 2003 and the question itself does not exist in a vacuum devoid of reference. That being stated the human noetic on an ascending trajectory and its motion of machinery is often not prone to acquiescence.

I often see great athletes with chronic lifetime disabilities from their sport when asked if they would do it again and most of the time I hear a "Yes" answer. Whether they truly feel that way when the television lights go out and they return home is questionable, if not fanciful. It is not beyond the perimeter of possibility that they often do not. Junior Seau the great NFL linebacker committed suicide at age 43 suffering from chronic traumatic encephalopathy (CTE). This diagnosis has appeared in other autopsy reports of the present- day gladiator. He died of a self- inflicted gunshot wound to the chest preserving the evidence found at autopsy. Chicago Bear great Dave Duerson did the very same one year earlier in 2011. A lawsuit is pending. A superannuated Earl Campbell, Heisman Trophy winner from the University of Texas and NFL Hall of Fame Houston Oiler is barely recognizable today. Depression, a multitude of surgeries, chronic pain, drug and alcohol abuse, as well as suicidal ideations followed his meteoric career. I sense his faith and family sustains him today. The awe we collectively felt for one Muhamad Ali in his prime has devolved into empathetic pity on gazing upon his caducity and empty eyes. The champ is no doubt still struggling as are countless others. One wonders if "The Greatest" even realizes how much he is struggling. There is something about youthful obduracy, money, power, and fame that at times produces a lachrymose short-sightedness, but that in part defines youth I think.

After Mr. Bloom's death there was as there always is a public surge of information regarding their disease. I believe his wife was very proactive in trying to bring VTE to the forefront. I also think that the fervor has since dramatically assuaged. Boston Red Sox manager Terry Francona had a pulmonary embolism the year his team won the World Series and had enlisted baseball legends to get the word out. It got out but it didn't stay out. Mr. Bloom went a perfect 3 for 3 on the Rudolf Virchow score card and never made it back to home plate. Time, international conflicts, and a severe monetary crisis produced a national fugue that obliterated other issues of weightiness.

It sadly appears that we are all stuck at first base without a shot of making it to second unless things radically change. Months after David Bloom's untimely death, pulmonary embolism had returned to the tenebrous shadows.

CHAPTER VIII

CHRONICLES (2) THE CASE OF THE BIZARRE LAST CZAR

IN THIS CHAPTER we will deal with the antipodal pathological end of the coagulation cascade which is when there is not a sufficient thrombus to be found. We leave Iraq and travel to Mother Russia.

The Romanov dynasty came to power in the 16th century after Ivan the Terrible met his maker. Probably the best recognized of this clan were "The Greats"- Peter the Great and Catherine the Great. Eventually Czar Nicholas II came to power and was given the avuncular title "Uncle Nicky." The detached lens of history nearly a century after his regency does not shine so kindly on this monarch who lacked dynamism and engineered his own tragic demise. His legacy is comparably invisible. He eventually married

Alexandra Feodorovna, winced accent and all, who was Hessian and was never loved by the Russian people. This was especially so since their country was at war with Germany in a little squabble called World War I. She was fertile though bearing the Czar five children. They were Olga, Tatyana, Maria, Anastasia, and the heir to the crown, Tsarevich Alexei.

What does this history have to do with the coagulation cascade? Alexandra was the carrier of hemophilia and it appears the source was her enate grandmother, none other than the sexually repressed Queen Victoria. Scientists believe it was the Queen Mother who developed the spontaneous mutation.

Unfortunately The Tsarevich was born with hemophilia and thus doted upon especially by a hovering Tsarina. It was the Alexandra's reliance on Grigori Rasputin an obsessed baffling religious figure, psychic, licentious womanizer, and faith healer that helped end the Romanov Empire. Rasputin was thought to have the power to heal Alexei and became a personal advisor to the monarchy. Nicholas II believed Rasputin when he induced him to believe that his empire could win the Great War. The Russian Revolution would have progressed without him just fine but his alliance to the crown just added to the unpopularity of Nicholas and Alexandra. Rasputin was eventually murdered a few months before the government coup. He professedly was not an easy kill as legend has it that he was rather mobile after some concoction of cyanide and bullets.

The 19th century was a tumultuous time period in Europe whose roots sprouted from The French Revolution. Reactionaries such as Karl Marx, Rosa Luxemburg, Nicholai Lenin, Leon Trotsky, Theodor Herzl, among a host of others were becoming increasingly prominent. They would eventually be more popular after World War I fearing the clear winner of the great conquest, the capitalistic United States. They were not wrong. Little did they know that after the next world war with the Roman numeral II following it, America would metamorphose into a bigger colossus. The destruction of German and Japanese global competition along with the Wall Street funding of Allied loans were two major reasons.

Prior to America's growth spurt the Industrial Revolution and the birth of Zionism helped foment labor movements from East to West. Amplified by the conflict to end all conflicts, famine, plagues, and a burgeoning new world order, it is plain to see the potential for regime change. It would be highlighted by the social cataclysm in Russia. The "Great" and the" Terrible" Tsars and Tsarinas were forever gone.

As a little boy the Tsarevich knew he would not live a normal life. His sister Olga found him lying on his back gazing at the supernal skies and asked him what he was doing. The child responded "Oh, so many things." "I enjoy the sun and the beauty of summer as long as I can. Who knows whether one of these days I shall not be prevented from doing this?" His words were eerily prescient. Nobody that young should be able to see the dark side that clearly.

Much more is understood about hemophilia now than it was in Alexei's time. Hemophilia is a sex-linked X chromosome disorder. In mammals the female has two X chromosomes, while the male has one X and one Y chromosome. Genes on X or Y chromosomes are called sex-linked. In fact it was not till recently that DNA proved he had hemophilia B which if recalled from that "Foolish" mnemonic he was deficient in factor IX, the Christmas factor. The other more prevalent hemophilia is hemophilia A where there is a deficiency in factor VIII. Hemophilia A is present in about 1 in 5000-10,000 male births. Hemophilia B is found in 1 in 20,000-34,000 male births. Males are more commonly affected since females have two X chromosomes and males only have one so a defective gene is guaranteed to manifest in the male carrier. People with hemophilia do not necessarily bleed faster or with more verve but they bleed longer. Often they will bleed into their joints especially the knees, elbows, and ankles. Hemarthrosis is the medical terminology. They can also bleed into their muscles and vital internal organs. Children with mild to moderate disease as defined by the amount of the deficient coagulation factor may not exhibit any early signs unless they are circumcised. As time goes on simple falls usually will produce bruising and hematomas (blood bubbles). The bleeding into the joints is especially painful. Effective treatment for the disease was not developed until the 1960s. Before that the life expectancy for a child was around 11 years of age. Today the average span is shorter by 10 years compared to the unaffected.

Needless to say Alexei was not allowed to participate in those activities that other boys were. Pastimes like rough-housing, bicycle riding, and sledding were prohibited. One can only imagine the toll it took on the youngster's psychology and it is not surprising that he intuitively knew his life would be truncated. Rasputin often used hypnotism and herbs when the boy was feeling sick and in pain. In all probability the faith-healer helped the child by advising the Tsarina to keep the physicians away. Probably not bad advice in the early 1900s. I imagine a hundred years from now they will be saying the same about our docs.

The imperial family was arrested during the tumult and coup following the 1st of two revolutions in 1917. In February Czar Nicholas II abdicated. While in Siberia Alexei snuck onto a sled and rode it down the steps and injured his pelvis. He hemorrhaged badly and became quite ill so that he could not be moved with his family in April when they were transferred to Ekaterinburg under house arrest. Eventually he joined his family three weeks later but was wheelchair bound and would remain so till his death.

The Romanov dynasty officially ended in the hot crepuscular hours of July 17, 1918 when the Bolsheviks, luxuriating in pure violence assassinated the entire family. One of the last family members to die was incredulously the Tsarevich with the bleeding disorder who was in fact the last Czar of Russia as his father was slain first. Why did the others bleed to death before he did? It was found that sewn in his tunic (as well as the others) were diamonds that deflected the bullets. One last gaze into the final hours of the

304 year old imperial dynasty revealed that the miscreant Grigori Nikulin emptied his gun's chamber into the boy's head. The only survivor of that un-cauterized bloody evening was the dog Jemmy. Alexander was thirteen.

Before we leave the merciless tale, Queen Victoria's eldest grandson the last German Emperor (and King of Prussia) Kaiser Wilhelm II died in 1941 from none other than a pulmonary embolism. He was the 3rd cousin to Nicholas II. The two abdicated their respective thrones 20 months apart. If one does not mind a Jerry Seinfeld intonation-the two evidently were good at getting a job, they just were not good at holding on to a job. Historical irony I guess? It would seem the "bad blood" between the Russians, the English, and the Germans started antebellum. Please excuse the lazy transition.

Despite the last two examples of the coagulation cascade misfiring, it is truly an exceptional system maintaining a delicate equilibrium inside the mammalian circulatory system. It seems that those with bleeding disorders tend to become clinically evident earlier than those with clotting disorders which tend to be concealed a bit longer and sometimes permanently. All the more reason I think that we need to bring this issue to the limelight.

We have discussed provoked versus unprovoked pulmonary embolisms in a previous chapter. To simply review, a provoked episode occurs in a patient with an antecedent (within 90 days) and transient major clinical risk. Things like surgery, trauma, pronounced inactivity, pregnancy as well as hormone replacement are in this rubric.

An unprovoked episode occurs in a patient with no prior major potential, who are not on hormones and have active cancer, a family history of VTE, or thrombophilia. Another way to think about the difference in addition to the voluntary vs non-voluntary explanation on page 25 is that in the latter the underlying liableness is constant and in the former, it is not.

Before the Bolsheviks came to power Vladimir Ilyich Lenin penned a revolutionary political pamphlet entitled "What is to be done." His vision ultimately failed but ours cannot. Hopefully VTE will never produce the same death count of all those who died and continue to do so under Communistic regimes but it is time to be proactive so the numbers never gets close.

There appears to be a modicum of options we can perform to affect the course of unprovoked VTE but I think with learning and insight we are proffered more control over this category of potential killer.

Immobility such as that which is produced on long airplane trips, prolonged bed rest, and long car rides, as well as male and female hormone replacement will be discussed in an attempt to answer Lenin's haunting question.

Comrade Lenin also died from a clot. He had a cerebral vascular stroke, the 5th leading cause of death in our homestead. His demise set the stage for yet another monster, Josef Stalin. The borscht in Eastern Europe would get intensively sourer.

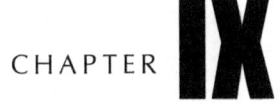

HOW DO YOU MAKE A HORMONE?

ONE OF THE most enigmatic topics in medicine since I graduated medical school has been the hormone estrogen. A hormone is a biochemical that influences physiology (function) and behavioral activities in living organisms. We apperceive from studies that the peril for myocardial infarction (heart attack) is lower for a woman than for a man till menopause and then it evens out. It is thought that estrogen protects the heart at least early on. But an unpalatable fact emerges when long term exposure to estrogen occurs, increased cardiovascular disease. The old glow was gone and the drug going forward would be crippled by its inconsistencies. Increased breast cancer, ovarian, and uterine cancer were all bruited about. There are accompanying factors such as age, family history, past medical history, the ratio of estrogen to another hormone progesterone, etc. that must be weighed. If articles are read from the 1980s, 1990s, and the 1st decade of the 2000s, the head begins to spin with the olio that emerges with varying recrudescent conclusions. A study thought inviolable one day was demolished the next. It seems that during the early menopause a little estrogen is good but if it outstays its welcome it can have deleterious effects. It has been a tedious irritation to many a healthcare provider and I have an aching sense that it will continue to be.

Of course one of them that is germane to this subject is its propensity to produce clots. Retrospective and prospective studies have shown a twofold to fourfold increase in the relative danger of VTE with its use. Some have shown up to 6 fold. In the Leiden Thrombophilia Study, the absolute odds for VTE was .8 per 10,000 per year among non-users of hormones and 3 per 10,000 per year among users. About 5% of all white women have the factor V Leiden mutation. They have an 8 fold increased probability for VTE and if concomitantly taking hormones that measured jeopardy can go up to fifteen fold. This must be weighed against the benefits of hormonal contraception such as preventing unwanted pregnancies along with the treatment of uterine bleeding and ovarian cysts. Birth control pills are currently thought to reduce both ovarian and uterine cancers. That might change again. Nevertheless by denying these genetic carriers oral contraception one might be causing more harm. Pregnancy is a risk for VTE. The first reported case of birth control thrombosis was in 1961 when a nurse taking a high-dose estrogen oral contraceptive had a PE. By the

1970s lower doses of estrogen were introduced into the new contraceptive pills. Once again the decision to go on these pills should be individualized. To be fair to hormones there are other drug classes associated with thrombi. Antidepressants, anti-inflammatory medicines, and the previously mentioned anti-neoplastic (cancer) treatments have all been indicted but estrogen has had an uncomfortably close relationship with the thrombotic state.

Estrogen replacement and contraceptive drugs containing hormones commands a huge market and I believe will continue to do so. However even without any genetic mutations these drugs pose a special potential problem to a large segment of the population. Often when a practitioner prescribes these medicines he or she is looking at a risk reward ratio which essentially is a compromise, meaning that neither party is full of delight and gratulation. In another words does taking the drug statistically outweigh its inherent liability of not taking it? There is a lot of randomness in disease processes.

Thankfully because estrogen replacement has been around there is a lot of data though at times conflicting. The first time it was marketed as a drug in the United States was 1933. The drug was named Emmenin, not to be confused with rapper Marshall Mathers III known as Eminem. He was born 39 years later in 1972. Emmenin was made from the human urine of pregnant Canadian females which was costly. In 1942 a patent was granted to Ayerst pharmaceuticals. Their product called Premarin would replenish the low levels of estrogen in women. Their product was made by extracting estrogens from pregnant horse urine. The name Premarin stands for **PRE**gnant **MAR**es' ur**IN**e. By 1977 when Eminem was 5 years old Premarin was the 5th most prescribed drug in America with more than 30 million prescriptions written. By the 1990s it was the most prescribed. By 2004 sales plummeted as studies started showing possible side effects of thrombi, heart disease, and cancer.

Female hormone replacement therapy (HRT) continues today in many forms. In fact the politically correct name is hormonal therapy and even lower doses are being produced now. Early studies on postmenopausal estrogen therapy showed a slight increased propensity for VTE. Subsequent studies were not as convincing but more recent studies done in the 1990s demonstrated a twofold to fourfold increase of venous thrombosis. As with birth control pills the opportunity for VTE is highest in year one of use. Women on hormone replacement who have the factor V Leiden mutation have a 15 fold increased risk of VTE. Data regarding the prothrombin 20210A mutation is meager. Sometimes these medicines are combined with other drugs and there is now a non- hormonal treatment for hot flashes.

Selective estrogen receptor modulators (SERMs) such as the drugs Tamoxifen and Evista (raloxifene) have anti-estrogenic effects and are used for the treatment of breast cancer and the prevention and treatment of osteoporosis. The MORE (Multiple Outcomes for Raloxifene) trial reported a 2 fold increase or greater chance of having a VTE with this drug class.

In general most healthy post -menopausal women would do well with some estrogen. It helps relieve dyspareunia (painful intercourse) due to vaginal dryness and promotes bone, cardiac, and mental health. Prior to starting the hormone some premonitory tests should be done like a lipid (cholesterol/triglycerides) profile and baseline liver function tests, including a thorough history and physical along with a mammogram. Some gynecologists order a preliminary pelvic ultrasound to ascertain the integrity of the uterus if present. I would argue that a screen for thrombophilia should accompany the aforementioned tests especially with a personal or family history of VTE and possibly without. Screening for patients without those histories is not recommended. I am not sure if I agree with that fiat as there are a lot of moving parts to entertain. It appears that the medical profession and the public are at least aware of the controversial and sometimes confusing hormone estrogen and its side effect profile. That is a good thing.

Unfortunately testosterone does not have the same data base. Male hypogonadism (men with low testosterone) generally meandered on unrecognized unlike the female menopause. Early studies on testosterone replacement were quite favorable. Men with lower levels it was reported had increased obesity, increased diabetes, increased lipids, were depressed more, had lower libidos, lower self-esteem, and were at higher risk for heart disease. Simply replenish the body with the testosterone anodyne and all will be well. Occam's razor is however double edged.

Unfortunately since the advent of the Low T (testosterone) syndrome, prescriptions for testosterone sky-rocketed and with that reports of deep vein thrombosis, pulmonary embolisms, and just in November 2013 in the Journal of the American Medical Association (JAMA) a reported increase in cardiovascular disease. The study has since been questioned. The reason seems to be that testosterone goes through a chemical reaction producing estrogen-like compounds in the body and they appear to be the primary culprits. Once again when more and more people are placed on a drug, more and more side effects appear. Some life threatening.

Just like with the long anfractuous history of estrogen, some drug trials are suggesting no increased propensity for VTE with exogenous testosterone. My sense is that there will be studies on both sides of the ovaries and testicles for many years.

As of this date the Food and Drug Administration has yet to punch the clock with a warning regarding testosterone therapy and venous thrombosis. Quite frankly I believe it is only a matter of time that they will once more data becomes available.

How does one make a hormone (whore moan)? The mordant answer to the lurid question used to be "don't pay her." I think the real answer is "carefully" and judging by the recent surge of class action lawsuits against the makers of pharmaceutical testosterone, "cautiously" may be the better riposte.

CHAPTER

AIR TRAFFIC out of CONTROL

COSMOLOGIST, AUTHOR, NATURAL science guru, astronomer, astrobiologist, and astrophysicist Carl Sagan once criticized a fellow scientist by saying that he had "impatience with ambiguity." I tend to listen to those requiring numerous commas when asked "What do you do for a living?" There are some who feel that the absence of evidence is evidence of absence. Others suggest that absence of evidence is not evidence of absence. Nevertheless there appears to be some connection between long flights and VTE. NBA star Chris Bosh and Haitian President Michel Martelly are among the many who developed pulmonary embolisms after recent air travel. Air flight may have presented an opportunity for some of the celebrities mentioned in the chapter 12 for whom clots developed. After all professional athletes are constantly in the air as are television/movie stars, sportscasters etc.

The current studies on VTE and air travel seem to be

producing mixed results. What else is new as the association between the two was first reported in the 1950s. The Centers for Disease Control (CDC) noted two studies reporting an absolute chance of a VTE for flights greater than 4 hours is 1 in 4656 flights and 1 in 6000 flights. It should be noted however that most passengers taking long flights are generally healthier and are not as exposed as the general population. Long-distance air travel may increase VTE by 2 to 4 fold. A similar danger seen by other modes of transportation. The Virchow factor of venous stasis appears to play a major role. Some studies have shown that 75%-99.55% of passengers who developed a VTE had one or more risk factors. However as previously discussed an inherited thrombophilia often asymptomatically lays in wait.

People who are less than 5 ft. 3 inches or greater than 6 foot 3 inches have a greater probability due to increased popliteal (behind the knee) pressure and less leg room respectively. Airline seats are generally not adjustable. The American College of Chest Physicians in 2012 published guidelines for long-distance travelers with a clotting propensity. They include frequent ambulation, calf muscle exercise, aisle seats if feasible, and the use of properly fitted below-knee graduated compression stockings that provide 15-30 mm of Hg (mercury) pressure at the ankle. These stockings were not recommended for those without risk factors nor were aspirin or anticoagulants. In one study window seats were reported to increase the chance of a bloody amalgam by 2-fold and in obese patients 6 fold. Needless to say it is difficult to officially register a controlled study in attempting to prove correlation yet alone cause and effect. There is a difference between the two from a statistical standpoint.

A simple example of a correlation versus cause and effect is the following. A rooster wakes up and makes a whole bunch of annoying noise. Soon afterwards the sun rises in the eastern sky. Farmers have been betting on that event sequence for years and have a perfect win-loss record. Despite that correlation if every rooster tomorrow contracted laryngitis and could not cackle I am willing to wager the empyreal blue would be illuminated anyway. The heavenly body could care less about the rooster. On the other hand if we reverse the scenario there is both correlation and cause and effect. Soon after the sun rises the next morning the rooster always cackles. Tomorrow our sun implodes. Say goodbye to the gallinaceous bird, their consulting throat doctors, and every edacious bookie who was willing to take action on the rooster. One day I think it will be proven that the connection between air travel and VTE is more than an aleatory.

It appears that at lofty altitudes the humidity is very low. There is some research suggesting that the body increases the level of clotting factors at around 8000 feet (oh that pesky diagram 1). Certainly seat-edge pressure on the popliteal area may cause vessel wall damage and stasis. Although I am not much of a traveler I have been on long flights neither drinking a sufficient quantity of fluids nor using the bathroom in a timely fashion. Dehydration, prolonged sitting, and low humidity unfortunately are all very thrombus friendly. Throw in the diuretic effect of alcohol, caffeine and certain medicines, along with certain hormones and the provoking dice are thrown. Officially the youngest woman on record dying from a PE after a long flight who was on birth control pills was a mere 28 years old.

I learned this from a fascinating article entitled "Prevention of Air Travel Blood Clot Fatalities" by Donald Daniel. An article that originated in 2004 and revised in 2013. The author lost a dear friend from a "flight induced PE" and feels the "airline industry would rather not admonish people of this danger for fear of scaring off customers." Is there any surprise that the Airport Transportation Associations general counsel, David Berg in 2003 said "In our view there is no direct relationship between air travel and deep vein thrombosis?" Wassup D.B. watering any artificial plants lately? A bit snippy and unimaginative don't you think? Dr. Sagan would not be pleased Dave.

I remember as a child seeing the numerous television commercials for tobacco companies. Salem, Lucky Stripe, Parliament just to name three. Big Tobacco's advertising budget was huge and they fought discolored tooth and nail to prevent the perilous possibilities from becoming discerned regarding the "vile weed." The image of the rough and tough macho quixotic Marlboro Man with his dedicated steed riding off in the sunset with a lit cigarette was etched in all our collective consciousness.

This gimmick in my humble opinion is another example of the Winston Churchill quote that "Truth is so precious that it is often accompanied by a bodyguard of lies." Perhaps Mr. Berg was just being a corporate obscurantist? He no doubt was responding to an ill-conceived lawsuit brought against the airline industry, but there is an inherent irresponsibility to that statement. We must always be wary of the unexamined assumption but to simply turn a blind eye to a red flag is infinitely more dangerous especially when buttressed by the strong lobbyists of our nation's airline industry.

Cause and effect or just correlation? It has been suggested that issued death certificates and airplane passenger ticket records be compared. If the traveler died within two weeks of flight for whatever reason it should be placed in a data bank. Low humidity must be maintained in aluminum skin planes due to water condensation but can be increased in those made of carbon fiber. Boeing is looking into increasing cabin humidity in their planes.

It is a start in the right direction but we must all be on lookout for those purveyors of half-truths and prevarications. I suspect the board rooms of the airline and tobacco industry bear a striking verisimilitude to each other.

Cigarette anyone?

CHAPTER XI

FIENDS, GENES, SCREENS, and CLINICAL SCENES

WELL WHAT IS to be done and what can be done are two different issues? I think Comrade Lenin was also aware of the quandary. What we know that cannot be done at least right now is to change our biological genome and from the prior chapters it is rather pellucid that hypercoagulable states are in most cases genetic as some are acquired.

Genetic testing and who pays for it is a very hot- button issue closely related to the politically fueled stem cell research and abortion debates. Already there are genetic tests that can be performed at home but there have been some quality control issues with these kits. Insurance companies armed with one's genetic profile may choose not to insure someone or manipulate the premiums. In my view religious and moral narratives will always be on the fringe and in general tend to provide an atmosphere of obfuscation.

What is the human brio worth? That answer depends on to whom that query is posited. Speak to a priest, a rabbi, an imam, or anyone representing an untainted entity and one would get a somewhat somber answer. Their reply would probably include a word meaning *sacrosanct* and something along the lines that one cannot put a price tag on one of G-d's creatures. Speak to a furtive insurance company executive and after a swift phone call to his or her actuaries, armed with certain demographic data you would get an answer down to the penny. It is a cold memorandum.

In a perfect world everybody would be mass screened for everything if so desired and then of course we as a society are left with the question as to whom will pay for all of it. Total body scans thickened the medical atmosphere for a few years but eventually disillusionment set in. People with means would pay big bucks to have their entire corpus imaged with the newest radiological imaging. The problem was that it would pick up things that many times were clinically insignificant, but to the patient with positive findings often an expensive goose chase ensued because of fear.

Another scenario in reference to genetic testing is what will the individual do with the information? Let's us say one has a gene associated with Alzheimer's disease. There is an APOE E gene found on chromosome 19 that may tip the scales towards getting the disease. Let us say one is 18 years old. Will that change anything for the adolescent armed with that knowledge? I don't think so. Right now one cannot do anything about it and I would imagine this could produce a negative psychological effect as was seen with the Tsarevich Alexei Nikolaevich. Although I am entrenched in the belief that in life not enough input is worse than too little, too much information can cause an anxiety producing white noise about findings that ultimately may have no clinical impact.

Another item to consider is the ever exigent uncertainty. We are schooled that if one smokes and drinks in excess, ingests foods laden with carbohydrates as well as fats, and leads a sedentary life that one's chances of dying early are increased. That behavior does not guarantee an early demise however. I would often have a soft-headed if not illusory medical student or two fumble through a story that they had some uncle who smoked 2 packs of cigarettes a day, drank a bottle of wine daily, had a pastrami sandwich for breakfast, drove his automobile blindfolded, and lived to 98. I always inquired if he did all those idiotic behaviors while simultaneously driving. These relatives were in reality outliers. Statistically a person is much better off doing the opposite. Personally I would move up the daily pastrami sandwich to lunchtime. With all due respect to the sanguine medical students I think some of them were merely launching a trial balloon well aware of the arrow that would soon deflate it. Also just because he lived to 98 he might have been chronically short of breath, on a ton of medicines including oxygen, and was a burden to other family members since he was 68.

My simple response to these Rhodes scholars and patients who felt the same way was this, if a blind man and a man with perfect vision were crossing a busy street which individual has a better chance making it to the other side unscathed? Of course the man with sight but the blind man could make it also. Ironically the man with the clear vision could get killed because he was concentrating on the recently recalled GM car but he did not see the Volkswagen with the elevated emissions. Entropy can be frustrating but it is rarely is it taciturn.

When studies are done in medicine the scientists look for outcomes and hopefully results occur that lead to certain recommendations that can reduce the chances of getting sick and dying early. We understand that a diabetic whose glucose is better controlled will probably have less complications than the diabetic whose blood sugar isn't. Most of what we grasp about heart disease originated from the Framingham Study that compared variables like cholesterol, blood pressure, age, tobacco use, body weight, glucose, etc. The term *evidenced based medicine* was derived from evidence discovered by trials. There are times these studies are flawed or repeat studies do not agree with the previous. Some studies materialize with surprises. Viagra was initially studied for coronary artery disease. It did not help the heart but the male participants noted differences in their erections. Hard to believe! Fish oil, Niacin, NSAIDS (non-steroidal anti-inflammatory drugs), E-cigarettes, and Vitamin D usages are controversial now because of newer studies. Studies on coffee seem to make the nightly news monthly. Fish oil has been recently shown to perhaps increase a man's possibility of getting a more aggressive prostate cancer. Niacin though it may improve a cholesterol profile may not change mortality. In another words one dies at the same age with a better cholesterol reading. Some academics swear by the need for Vitamin D especially for those with limited exposure to the sun (Vitamin D production is modulated by solar exposure). Vitamin D is good for bone, cerebral, and cardiovascular health. Some think that it may help prevent autism. Others eschew that the Vitamin D craze is overblown and unwarranted. Even aspirin, one of our most time-tested and beloved drugs is under review as there is some evidence, anecdotal perhaps that there is a link between its use and pancreatic cancer. The FDA in 2015 is now warning the public about Aleve, Motrin, and the rest of the drugs we use for aches and pains due to its cardiovascular effects in some people. In the same year proton pump inhibitors like Prilosec, Prevacid, and Nexium that are used to protect us from getting ulcers and control acid reflux may also be linked to heart and kidney disease. Ironically they are often used when taking the aforementioned NSAIDS to protect the lining of our gastrointestinal tracts.

The electronic cigarette (E-cigarette) use has tripled amongst teens from 2013-2014. The battery powered vaporizer simulates the feeling of smoking and is supposed to be the next chiliastic product in regards to tobacco cessation. The brickbats from the medical community too have tripled as ongoing investigations are producing some unfavorable results. It may be our domain's next vexatious addiction for profit as the studies regarding its safety and efficacy are all over the map similar to the hormone studies. Coffee has a long history of being culpable from stunting growth to causing cancer and heart disease. Other studies suggest that it helps prevent diabetes, liver disease, and neurodegenerative maladies like Parkinson's and Alzheimer's.

Another problem is us, our cellular identity. We all have special genes. One person can take a drug to prevent stroke and it works well because they do not burn the drug up so quickly. In another words it remains in their circulation the "proper" time. Others metabolize the medicine at such an excessive pace that it is eliminated briskly leaving the patient vulnerable. Others cannot metabolize fast enough so they have too much circulating thus increasing the risk of hemorrhage. With all the drugs and all the genes it is impossible to give a patient a 51% guarantee yet alone a 100%. Look at any drug side effect profile or the way an individual awakens from general anesthesia (also a drug) or reacts to a vaccination and one is immediately struck by the variance of humanity. It is an interesting proxy for our heterogeneous genetic makeup.

Because of their popularity diseases like diabetes, heart disease, cancer, and asthma have had many studies and are continuing. There have been studies regarding VTE. The PIOPED Study (Prospective Investigation of Pulmonary Embolism Diagnosis), the previously alluded to Worchester DVT study, the 2013 MOPETT TRIAL (Moderate Pulmonary Embolism Treated with Thrombolysis), the European PEITHO study (Pulmonary Embolism Thrombolysis), and the TOPCOAT study (Treatment of Sub-massive Pulmonary Embolism with Tenecteplase or Placebo: Cardiopulmonary Outcomes at Three Months) are just some. The last two were looking at the efficacy and safety of thrombolytic drugs, particularly Tenecteplase, in the treatment of sub-massive pulmonary embolisms. If the results can be substantiated that patients with a moderate pulmonary embolism seem to improve faster with thrombolytic drugs once used for only the unstable patient then treatment protocols may be modulated in the future. The general medical community has thus far given that idea a cool reception as the serious problem of intracranial bleed increases with its use. Only time and tough scholarship will determine if it remains a crooked gear or waxes into a mechanism with less of a coefficient of friction.

However unlike a genetic test that shows one may be at risk for Alzheimer's, the screening tests for thrombophilia could provide data to impact the person's decision making in hopes of lowering their chance of VTE at any age. So all genetic tests are not created equally.

Also at risk for VTE are people with anatomical variants that unlike in those with thrombophilia, are seen macroscopically either by imaging or surgically. They too are essentially genetic at their core. Examples are the May-Thurner syndrome in which the veins in the lower leg are compressed by an overlying artery and the congenital absence of the inferior vena cava. I include them for completion sake only. They are exceedingly rare and not subject to any screening protocol.

So should all people be screened for all things? Not in this world for as Benjamin Franklin once quipped "We are all obliged to the economy." I do envision one day that smart phones will have the ability to hold our personal genome and our screened tests in one storage file as will smart governments. What is done with the information is the question.

But should some people be screened for some things? The answer is yes and that is being done already for less protean illnesses. We screen for diabetes, high cholesterol, sickle cell, breast cancer etc. The list goes on. Should people tabula rasa (blank slate) be screened for these genetic hypercoagulable states? I would argue no, but yes for certain subsets of our society especially those with an equivocal family or personal history of excess clotting. That history is not often obvious and requires some digging that often borders on excavation. Some slates appear blank because the right queries were not asked or the wrong ones were. A physician's index of suspicion must be continually honed.

How about for example a pilot on exogenous testosterone who is responsible for getting passengers from the United States to Vietnam. That is a good 17 hours of sitting. His father and uncle both had strokes in their 40s. Consider the truck driver who is traveling hours on end without a stop and has a vague recollection of a painful swollen calf that resolved on its own? He is not the type to run to doctors. How about the gallivanting business woman on Premarin who has had 3 "unexplained" miscarriages and smokes.

Her doctor has since died and she has no idea where her medical records are. How about a 51 year old experiencing menopausal flashes whose general practitioner thinks she might have lupus. Her gynecologist recommended estrogen replacement but she cannot afford the copay to see a rheumatologist at the current time. She never boards a plane but drives a municipal bus on the weekdays and likes to play hours of bingo on the weekend? How about the youngster on birth control pills who flies cross-country to college? She remembers her half-sister was once hospitalized for "some kind" of clot in her lung or was it asthma? They have lost touch with each other since their dad remarried. How about a middle-aged obese man who is attached to the "bottle" with a desk job for whom topical testosterone was prescribed. He has a "weird" history of a possible clot in his abdomen but the doctors couldn't prove it? They just warned him about alcohol causing liver disease. How about anyone who may have had a possible thrombus undergo testing? How about a reporter with "leg cramps" who is to be embedded with the US army and anchored to a vehicle's floor for hours in the desert heat?

I have nothing but dithyrambic praise for "evidenced base medicine" but should common sense be eliminated from judicious decision making? Many times in my practice I felt more like a dentist because getting an accurate history was like pulling teeth. It is not black or white but it can be life or death. Is it cost effective? My simple reply is yes and no and cost effective for whom? Every once in a while there is a new study or a rejuvenated old one that raises doubt about the wisdom of early breast cancer screening with mammography or prostate cancer screening with a blood test called a PSA (prostate specific antigen). Like the total body scans the screening does lead to further unnecessary tests, worry, and may or may not statistically reduce overall mortality. Logical perhaps but here is the dirty little secret, I am unaware of any of my physician coevals who do not get screened early for these potential killers. Furthermore when their progeny enter adulthood they also recommend, if not command them to do the same. It is like insider trading combined with a somewhat odd form of professional courtesy. Most professions treat their "own" a bit differently but there is too much at stake when dealing with people's health issues to always remain rigidly aligned to the medical recommendations de jour.

Despite population studies and protocols they are to be treated as guidelines, not immutable god-lines. With the advent of EHR (electronic health records) though still in its incunabula the ability to data collect is outstanding. As more and more computers whimsically talk amongst themselves along with smarter cell phones and tablets medical statisticians truly can feast on bigger and bigger digital repasts. Maybe one day the doctor will be able to hit a button and all will be known before the patient's blood pressure cuff deflates. I would not wager on it. For now fancy pie charts, colorful diagrams, pamphlets, recommendations and regulations will have to do. As discussed and to reiterate "facts" that looked important in 2010 may look impotent in 2014 and what was blown off as insignificant a few years back now may be in bold capital letters in the prestigious New England Journal of Medicine(NEJM). We as clinicians have to do a better job at asking the question "Why?" at a faster pace. It is a Sisyphean task as the increasing responsibilities placed upon physician's shoulders would not only make Atlas shrug but his knees to collapse. Bilateral titanium knee replacements are not the answer.

I would have been thrown out of my internship in 1982 if I would have treated a patient in congestive heart failure (CHF) with a beta blocker (drug class) as it was totally contraindicated. Currently it is the drug of choice for patients suffering from the same.

I think most people look at science as a homogenous discipline but it is anything but. I would doubt that one can find a physicist today who would wager that Newton's Three Laws of Motion will change in 100 years. In comparison I could not fathom a physician thinking that 10 years from now the model, monitoring, and treatment of cardiovascular disease, cancer, and asthma just to name 3 will be the same. As I was writing this chapter The American Cancer Society has once again changed their guidelines for breast cancer screening with mammograms. The American College of Radiology has not. Don't get me wrong there are plenty of tenets in medicine that I do believe will hold serve. Certainly if a patient is dehydrated then fluids is the treatment along with trying to figure out as to why the person is desiccated. Makes sense right, but 200 years ago the best physicians were doing the exact opposite. They were bleeding the "ill humors" from their sick dehydrated patients making them more parched. President Washington who probably had tonsillitis or a syndrome called quinsy, which is an abscess around the tonsils probably died from the procedure.

One needs only to tune in to CNBC and listen to those with PhDs in the science of economics trip over their predictions as to where interest rates are heading or what the dollar-yen ratio will be. Quite frankly if the American Heart Association and the American College of Cardiology once again changes the guidelines for the treatment of elevated cholesterol in an attempt to reduce cardiovascular mortality I am going to have a heart attack. Rarely in the practice of medicine is anything both certain and true over the long run. There indeed is some veracity to the statements "There are lies, damn lies, and statistics" and "Do as I say not as I do." The bottom line is that not all of science is created equally as is manifested in genetic testing.

However in today's science the mortality and morbidity of thrombo-embolic disease is not in doubt and it is imperative that screening be afforded some wiggle room. Patients simply do not always have a grasp on their family history or theirs for that matter. Doctors simply do not have the luxury to dig deep into these histories due to time restraints. Therefore if something sounds like there could have been some abnormal clotting mechanism involved then the bar must be set a tad lower. Better to err on the side of prudence. The CEO of the multimillion dollar insurance company will surely understand and it is really too damn bad if he or she doesn't. With that expansion the

healthcare professional and consumer will be better educated as to what possibly lurks within.

When the heavily made up weather-woman on television warns us of potential flooding, heavy snows, high
winds etc. viewers usually respond to the warning. They
make sure they have boots, umbrellas, flashlights, shov-
els, battery operated radios. People might tie down their
patio furniture, purchase sandbags, buy a generator with
instructions made for Mensa members, and take further
precautions depending on the forecast. If the pattern is severe enough like an oncoming tornado, hurricane, or tsu-
nami the municipal, state, and federal governments may
get involved. Why would anyone not want to recognize a
possible impending disaster if the winds within them are
pointing that direction? At least one can make sure that
one is adequately hydrated; that one is not planted in a
single position for hours; that one's clothing is not so tight
that blood flow is obstructed; that one's legs are not compressed against the edge of the seat; that if one is having surgery then the surgeons and anesthesiologists are
warned about the propensity to have exuberant clotting.

At least armed with a cellular understanding a person
would have in essence a molecular "informed consent" as
to what medicines to go on and the risk/reward ratio of being on them. Additionally they would be more cognizant
of early symptoms that under normal circumstances may
be disregarded as nothing.

With that stated thrombophilia screening should not
be overused as anticoagulants which are replete with

ridiculous expense and life-threatening complications would be over-prescribed. Additionally patients could be defined by a disease that has no present or future clinical impact. Issues like life insurance eligibility and disability are just two of many possible needless headaches.

You cannot swim outside your gene pool but by understanding the depth in depth, one can in some cases swim for longer distances measured in years. Why be found dead in the water because of ignorance or negligence?

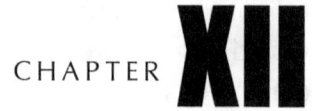

WHAT is to be DONE?

VTE HAS AFFECTED some well-known people. Terry Francona, Kaiser Wilhelm, and David Bloom are just a blood-drop in the bucket. Here are some others.

Tennis great Serena Williams.

NBA Cleveland Cavalier star Anderson Varejao.

Stacy Andrews of the NFL had his career ended during week 13 of the 2011 season.

Derrick Thomas superstar for the NFL Kansas City Chiefs after sustaining paralyzing injuries in a motor vehicle accident died weeks later from a massive PE age 33.

Celebrity hair stylist Annabel Tollman died age 36.

TV host Regis Philbin had a thrombus in his leg removed at age 78.

Actress Zsa Gabor at age 93 developed a PE.

Professional golfer Joey Sindelar in 2009 became dizzy and short of breath while playing at the Charles Schwab Cup Championship. He was diagnosed with a PE at age 51.

Actor Jimmy Stewart died of a PE at age 89.

NASCAR driver Brian Vickers developed a DVT/PE at age 26.

Major league baseball player 1st baseman for the Boston Red Sox Harry Agganis died at age 26.

Musician Heavy D dead at age 44. Originally thought to be a complication of pneumonia. Craig Harvey, head of the Los Angeles County Department of Coroner stated that the blood clot that resulted in a PE was "most likely formed during an extensive airplane ride." He had recently returned from Wales.

NBA star Chris Bosh missed half of the 2014 season after complaining of fatigue and side pain. Further tests would reveal multiple pulmonary emboli. He had flown to Haiti just prior.

Assassin Jack Ruby sentenced to death by a lethal pulmonary embolism secondary to lung cancer.

American tenor and Hollywood star Mario Lanza died after a hospital stay to lose weight age 38.

Comedienne Totie Fields died at 48.

Thacher Longstreth, the ultimate WASP Philadelphia Councilman died at age 82. Blue-blood indeed.

Dan Blocker TV Bonanza star died from a post-operative PE.

Richard Nixon a month after resigning the Presidency of the United States in 1974 developed a DVT. No lie.

Tenor Placido Domingo was hospitalized for a PE at age 72 while in Spain.

Detroit Mayor and ex- NBA star Dave Bing was

hospitalized for a PE, released, and had to return the same week. Back on the foul line.

Haiti's president Michel Martelly at age 51 had a PE two weeks after surgery. He had flown to Florida post-operatively.

Actor Dennis Farina died from a PE at age 69

NBA star Jerome Kersey died of a PE days after knee surgery. Age 52

Bonnie Bernstein superb sportscaster for ESPN and previously ABC went 2 for 2 as a DVT migrated to both her lungs. Multiple airplane trips, birth control pills, and a then unknown family history of blood clots rounded out the trifecta.

Steve Reeves the body builder-actor made famous for his portrayals of Hercules (once the highest paid screen star in Europe) died from a post-operative PE. A giant of a man cut down by a leviathan measured in mere millimeters.

NHL star Pascal Dupuis sat out 6 months from the 2014-15 hockey season due to a PE. This was his 2nd that was diagnosed. He was readmitted to the hospital for similar symptoms in the November 2015. The tests were negative. Sound familiar?

Along with Terry Francona major league baseball legends Tony Gwynn, Phil Niekro, Rolle Fingers, Paul Blair, Dennis Eckersley, Jim Fregosi, and Aaron Cook all of whom had been touched by DVT were involved with a campaign to educate the public beginning in 2004.

Ever hear them speak? I haven't. The list goes on and on. One would think with high profile people in high profile professions that the word would get out and stay out but it doesn't.

After the baseball New York Giants beat the Washington Senators in the 1933 World Series there was a huge add in the city's papers "21 of the 23 Giants World Champions Smoke Camels. It Takes Healthy Nerves to Win The World Series." Maybe the tobacco industry could use the Airport Transportation Association's attorney Mr. Berg and the Marlboro Man on Joe Camel for their next gig. Oh that's right they are not allowed anymore gigs but eight decades later the corporate rhetoric remains clamant and unclear. Perhaps the majority of multinational corporations tend to be dubious sponsors of the truth because it appears that inherent to advertising is the language of unrealistic absolutes. I have a wounding suspicion that will never change.

Unlike in mathematics there are no immutable proofs when dealing with the living. When dealing with biological organisms there are correlations, conclusions from studies with limited sampling pools, concealments, corollaries, and "evidences" that are not always carved in stone. Medicine which is replete with information and misinformation often provide an arbitrage opportunity for tricksters trying to make a quick profit. I am sorry to say that some of these hoaxers have medical degrees. The Christopher Hitchens quote rings true "That which can be asserted without proof can be dismissed without proof," but as John Adams said whilst defending the Redcoats in court "Facts are stubborn things."

I think in order to get the message to stay in the human

cerebrum then the modern day Perseus must take the form of government, Hollywood, sports, print media, corporations, public service announcements, religious institutions, charities, healthcare professionals, and social media. The recent Arab Spring was somewhat successful due to a large part because of engaged Facebook, Instagram, and Twitter users. The three sites and others could be important contributors to this rebellion also.

What a perfect segue way for every major league baseball's 7th inning stretch to have the announcer simply say "Move those legs get popcorn not clots." How about after the flight attendant brimming with synthetic politeness gives the perfunctory directions on how to put an oxygen mask on (when you are plummeting from 40,000 feet) reminds everybody to uncross their legs, intermittently wiggle their feet, and to drink plenty of water. At least put some kind of written warning on the seats.

It seems to me that the pharmaceutical industry who have been so immensely successful at selling their wares should simply include the indications of their drugs for VTE on the television commercials. It is interesting to note that the erectile dysfunction drug Cialis in larger doses is used to treat pulmonary hypertension, a complication of PE. Stay up and keep your pulmonary pressures down!

I think when Robert De Niro and a rather coxcomb looking Samuel L. Jackson advertise for American Express and Capital One credit cards respectively, the consumer listens. Comics just don't make us laugh, they make us think. Twenty years later people still remember the Seinfeld

Show and its themes as if it were yesterday. Could you imagine if Robert, Samuel, or Jerry did spots for this deadly disease along with other stars?

Hospitals, urgent care facilities, and clinics by placing posters for DVT prevention in their lobbies and elevators would help. During a recent hospitalization I was shocked as I thought I saw a sign that said "Avoid Clots!" When I put on my glasses the sign said "Avoid Clogs!" "Only Put Paper Products down the Toilet. No Feminine Napkins." Plumbers 1 Patients 0. In 2014 there were 4 laboratory confirmed cases of Ebola virus and 1 death in the United States yet hospital walls continue to be strewn with Ebola posters. Fear tends to make a more eye-catching wallpaper than fact.

How about on television and the big screen that people once in a while die from a pulmonary embolism and not the old-fashion heart attack? The NBA, MLB, NHL, and the NFL could bring this disease to the forefront while fans are sitting for hours on end watching the games (hopefully intermittently getting up). Not to mention college sports and their advertisers. I would watch "The Clot Bowl." How about during the annual college NCCA basketball series known as "March Madness" a [PE vs. DVT bracket] appears with the other 32 matchups. Contests that are highlighted in every major newspaper. Out of all the sport extravaganzas this forum would be the most apropos (final chapter will explain).

Russ Limbaugh on his radio show can say that VTE is a Democratic Party conspiracy theory, but at least his steady listeners would be made more aware as they attempt to wrest the cords of political power.

An occasional public service announcement on television and radio from the United States government would help. Certainly the Amyotrophic Lateral Sclerosis (ALS) campaign that went viral in the summer of 2014 where celebrities challenged other celebrities to be dumped with a bucket of ice cold water and be filmed, injected a huge infusion of cold cash for research. NBC could do an annual tribute to David Bloom.

In a step in the right direction the CDC has recently launched a program to honor healthcare facilities that have implemented effective strategies to prevent healthcare associated clots. It is called The "HA-VTE Challenge" and it is replete with prize monies and nonmonetary recognition for winning submissions. That would look good on a billboard?

Perhaps if state governments would replace one or two monthly lottery commercials with ads for VTE prevention, there would be more of us around to play their rigged game. Can't we find any room on the municipal buses to advertise? Surely there must be some space between the pictures of the smiling Afro-American attendee of that brand new online school and the company that takes your 30 year-old bathroom and converts it to a brand new one by gluing acrylic templates over your existing fixtures. Do they remove the pre-existing mold first? When that bright-eyed kid completes his Harvard-like education via laptop what are the financial terms of the loan he now needs to repay? 12 years a slave indeed and possibly longer.

The major health insurers have deep pockets and have recently increased their bets on preventive care. This disease screams to be heard. Sirius Radio has a station called "Doctor Radio" with a rather huge following including myself that could educate both healthcare professional and patient.

Just ads in magazines whose circulation (pun not intended) are geared to the young and athletic as well as those for the older segments like the AARP would help promote a bimodal national conversation not yet sustained.

Larry Kudlow an economist employed by the Reagan Administration and former host of "The Kudlow Report" on CNBC said every night "We believe that free market capitalism is the best path to prosperity." With that prosperity we should be able to allocate resources so that this disease gets its fair shake. So many of us are glued to our computers sitting for hours on end. A screen saver or a piece of software could remind us to get up and circulate our erythrocytes. Could an App be far behind? The mediocre actuarial effort put forth so far is beyond tragic. If *Medusa's Clot* has an edge to it there is a good reason, something needs to be done!!!!!

There are many websites but people have to recognize something before they begin a search. This disease has been allocated in a relative sense to the dustbin of history. Smallpox belongs there not DVT/PE.

The more people that understand the disease the more an individual can do, but unfortunately it is a short list in relative terms. Certain industries are not going to worry that their customer has been sitting for hours in one spot. Bartenders are not going to warn their besotted patrons that it is time to get up and move around. The movie theaters are not going to admonish their customers to stand up after two hours and obstruct the view of those sitting behind them. But make sure all cell phones are off. The gaming industry is not going to place placards on their machines and gaming tables stating *2 hour sitting limits*. Even if they did they would be as phony as the signs stating *Gambling Problem? - Call 1800 Gambler*. One would develop a clot and a migraine headache just waiting for the operator to answer.

Interestingly a recent published report about compulsive gambling linked the activity to anxiety, depression, fibromyalgia, migraine, irritable bowel syndrome, and other chronic illnesses. One day I fervently believe that thrombo-embolic disease will be on that list.

My ex-mother-in-law who appeared in excellent health and looked 20 years younger than her age died suddenly at a casino. It is indeed possible that she had a silent culprit lesion in a coronary artery but she may have very well had a massive pulmonary embolism causing the cardiac arrest. Sitting for hours in a low humidity environment and drinking dehydrating caffeinated beverages is as bad at a gaming hall as it is on a plane plus one has the additional factor of inhaling toxic cigarette smoke. She was all of 4 foot 9 inches tall, no doubt blood was pooling in her dangling lower extremities while her popliteal spaces were being compressed.

As individuals it is imperative that we keep well hydrated, move around, even wiggling our feet no matter how stupid we look. For G-d's sake uncross those legs!

If you want to stave off other chronic diseases like diabetes, heart disease, depression, obesity, and early death for a while just to name a few the following will help. Stay lean, drink alcohol moderately, exercise, wash your hands often, do not smoke, eat a Mediterranean type diet (fish, nuts, virgin olive oil, berries), drink plenty of water, wear seat belts, and MOVE even when you are feeling a tad lazy! As we lurch forward so does technology making us less civil and more stationary by degree. Computers, video games, pizza delivery, and spectator sports keeps us sitting. Fast food drive-ins supply us with excess carbohydrate and fat calories without us even having to exit our vehicles and burn a few up prior to ingesting their addicting fare.

Our hunter gatherer ancestors would have never imagined a world so replete with chairs and so devoid of physicality. They would take a lachrymose view with spears raised upon seeing both. We have at the same time evolved into such brilliance and devolved into such otiose stupidity. The opprobrium of our contemporary physically sedate lifestyle is as the Roberta Flack song says is "Killing us softly." If we are really unlucky it can kill us quickly especially if we inherited the wrong parents.

We can have an impact by modulating the 1st two-thirds of Virchow's Triad. The problem is the remaining third, that which causes hypercoagulable states and the not-so-funny business of genetics. For many people DNA stands for *Do Not Ask*. That is a not-so-curious mistake on many levels. One cannot escape their genes but by seeing the cards dealt one can at least take precautions and tip the odds in one's favor. Genetic testing should be expanded.

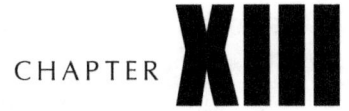

JUDGES
In G-D WE SHOULD PROBABLY TRUST:
ROLE of FAITH in DISEASE

ONE MIGHT ASK why is there a chapter about faith in a book devoted to the subject of pulmonary embolism. The Lord only knows how much I wrestled with its inclusion but with every book there is a thrombosed vein that requires opening. There were other considerations as stated in the following.

Faith along with mindfulness, acupuncture, tai chi, yoga, massage, supplements, etc. are getting a lot of traction in the integrative conversation about acute and chronic disease. Mind-Body centers are popping up throughout the United States and are increasing in popularity. When a person gets sick it is important that they have access to a toolbox containing various instruments, belief being one of them. Some of these utensils like supplements as an example may be a black box as they are not FDA approved but can provide benefit. The patient's toolbox which includes Western Medicine has, is, and will always be a work in progress.

The following sentence is not meant to be a lapidary phrase. Let me be perfectly clear that without my acceptance of a higher being there was a good chance that I would have been amongst the 41,000 people who take their own life annually. One might be reminded from page XII that suicide is the 10th leading cause of death in America (it is probably the 11th). I have been through a lot in my life and I have always been able to tough it out. This monster's clot came awfully close to taking me down the self-inflicted road which happens once every 13 minutes in this country. Without including this chapter I would not have been able to live with myself. Feeling that way once was enough. That avouched I think the four top obstacles to the common weal is climate change, nuclear proliferation, pathogenic organisms (bacteria, viruses, fungi, parasites), and radicalized religion with particular attention to Islam at this point in time. The 4th impediment may indeed be more infectious than the 3rd?

Thirdly why a chapter on belief in juxtaposition to illness? Many people have lost faith in many things once thought tried and true. Their government, their employers, their legal structure, their religious leaders, and their healthcare system which includes their healers just to name a few. Belief in something could provide some well needed support. More to follow as the subject requires more than an en passant paragraph.

In this "twist of lime" chapter I want the reader to understand that my views on this subject are intensely personal and in no way meant to offend anybody. This chapter is not for the play-it-safe crowd. I advance in suggestion only that there will be those who vehemently agree, those who violently disagree, and a slight few who will vigorously agree and disagree. Much of the following has been culled from decades of reading both atheistic and religious disquisitions with whatever enhancements I could add. The core philosophical arguments for and against faith have not changed radically over the years, merely burnished. I hope the long and diverse bibliography has provided me sufficient polish to increase the sparkle.

One accounting note, that when discussing historical figures it is all too common to point to their brainstorms and actions that have been ultimately proven wrong centuries later. Sapient hindsight can often be unfair and acidulated. As an example for years the world revolved around the science of Aristotle until challenged by Galileo. The great student of Plato was scientifically way off base but he should not be belittled for his 2500 year old insights. They were at the time based on the observational gestalt of the day. Anybody now who gives credence to the Aristotelian model is probably more often than not inebriated and should probably not be teaching science anywhere.

For those interested in only the tangible aspects of VTE and are secure in their beliefs then my best advice is to skip to page 185. For the multitude who wrestle with conviction, who want to believe but cannot find a pathway, it is my hope that a different road has been made manifest. It is not my intention for people to rethink their belief system. My desideratum is to give people who do not have a belief system but possibly desire one a viable alternative.

One last subject that we briefly touched upon above needs some elucidation before moving forward. No book on VTE is complete without a few paragraphs about the bureaucracy that dictates its management. A directorate with whom many have lost conviction.

Twenty years ago I wrote a book entitled *White Chocolate* which was about my medical career caring for the Afro-American community in Northwest Philadelphia. Actually it was my passion still very much alive. The publication has long since been out of print which is exactly where it should be. In those days however I was fortunate to have made a few appearances on television, radio, and in the city newspapers so the paperback sold rather well. It dealt with many topics but the one germane to *Medusa's* Clot was its chapter XIV entitled "Un-Managed Care-A Manifestation of a World Gone Awry." It was a poke at the rapidly changing medical bureaucracy that was then still in its relative early stages. The most expensive healthcare system per capita that treated health as a sick commodity. Two decades years later it is boundlessly expensive, profoundly unmanaged, and unbelievably ill despite sentient efforts to produce the obverse.

The American healthcare system, like most large technologically dependent complexes tends to marginalize patients over time, often reducing them to a mere digital entry in their electronic healthcare record (EHR). As consolidation continues that marginalization will be made worse as patients will feel more indisposed. The same words I wrote in 1996. Medicine has been reduced to a business model as more and more physicians become employees, and more and more employees become myrmidons. Bean counters, business people in fine outfits as well as new corporate logos will only increase as the relationship between doctor and patient will be efficiently made less embroidered. One wonders when Amazon will get involved in the distribution of care when house calls are performed by physicians and nurses escorted on drones and driverless cars. Google is now in the mortgage business as business boundaries continue to be breached.

I would think that technology would have made a court appearance by now. To a certain degree that would make more sense than a jury system steeped in emotion that is often moved by great orators and not great facts. Simply figure out fair and logical algorithms that defines "beyond a reasonable doubt" and other legal standards. Hit the red button after feeding in all the evidence, legal briefs, as well as testimonies and the probabilities of honesty vs culpability are printed out that can be reviewed by juries and judges. That of course will never happen as the legal racket unlike the medical profession knows how to fend for themselves.

My craft does not and has sold themselves out a long time ago. Patients who are sick do not have much of an emotional banister to hold on to nowadays. The crutches made in China and sold at Walmart won't do the trick either. There was a time when the general practitioner's office was a place where the infirmed could safely and confidentially moor. The days when the doctor's receptionist picked up the phone after one ring and knew the patient's voice on the other end are long gone. Her familiarity with the person's family is also in the recycle bin, emptied daily. Her boss crippled by procedural codes, regulations by both government as well as private payers, memorandum dictates from a central hub regarding efficiencies as well as outcomes, and increasing malpractice premiums have shackled their doctor. The beloved general practitioner (GP) - family doctor (FP)-primary care physician (PCP) is often aloof, robotic, and reduced to alphabet soup. To avoid confusion PCP is also the abbreviation for phencyclidine, affectionately known by some as the illicit recreational drug Angel Dust. Sadly physicians are more likely to misuse opiates than the general population according to Dr. Lisa Merlo, researcher at the University of Florida's Center for Addiction Research and Education. Depression and burnout are on the rise amongst American physicians and their suicide rates have been for years the highest in the nation. The reasons are multifactorial but the job itself has a lot to do with these crushing trends. It is difficult to care for others when one cannot care for oneself and a nation that cannot adequately care for its sick eventually cannot care for itself.

Today's physicians have their already busy lives dictated to in some form or another by board members, CEOs, government bureaucrats, accountants, and lawyers. All with their endless no-brainer opinions, tautologies, and proliferated attempts at certainty with their "ifs, ands, and buts." Let us not forget the word "wherefore." The new 2015 International Classification of Disease known as ICD-10 which are the billable diagnostic codes are as complex as the IRS rules and regulations. G-d forbid the physician does not check off the right boxes or omits a date on the encounter form. Somehow with all this the good doc needs to keep voraciously reading so to keep up with the burgeoning information on diseases and the new drugs on the market. Not to mention which insurance entity will and will not pay for them. Is this the proper time for a pungent utterance about attorneys and their litigious clients? The solo practitioner who once administered to the patient their childhood immunizations and years later their adult blood pressure medicines is but an oneiric fantasy. The physician with whom one counted on when the weathered wheels began to loosen is not the same often buried in a group of others. During the visit there is one eye on his (her) computer/tablet screen, one ear on the patient, one ear on the phone, and the other eye on the clock.

When one goes to the mega pharmacy drive-in to fill a prescription their facial recognition cerebral software is even worse. "How do you spell your name again?" "Oh that medicine needs a *prior authorization*, your doctor needs to send information to your insurance company so they will pay for it." The regulated primary care office is much too engaged for phone calls so the proprietorship installed the most up to date electronics for digital communiques. So now one emails the office or uses their fancy password protected Internet portal that allows a patient do just about anything, but speak to someone. Hopefully somebody gets the message, maybe the nurse practitioner (NP) or physician assistant (PA).

The local hospitals we knew are extinct or have coalesced with the bigger ones. The building is the same, the personality isn't and the vital signs just feel differently despite a certificate from the JCAHO (Joint Commission on Accreditation Health Organizations). It all feels so mawkish. If a patient is deemed sick enough some hospitalist will care for them. "What is your name again doc?" The general practitioner years ago gave up his "Doctors Only" parking card after the hospital was bought the 1st time. The sign on the edifice is its 3rd in 14 years. The primary care physician will get a letter regarding his patient's admission a week later which will be filed with the other thousand pieces of glimpsed-at mail. Is a glance a shorter period of time?

Don't get me wrong a Luddite I am not. The sinews of technology are wonderful but patients often feel lost and herded about without compass or rudder within its fibers. Most of the previous words, and they are meant to be taken as a generalized landscape only, primarily relates to the baby- boomers. The "awesome" generations X, Y, and Z and the ensuing "uninitialized" will know only the current reality. Maybe they are lucky as they won't have the opportunity to look back with a pardonable last yearning gaze. Unfortunately it is the aging segment of our population whose parts have been worn down by time and distance that needs the majority of the costly refurbishing.

So this chapter on belief is written for three reasons. To help with personal despair and isolation, to understand and perhaps make it easier for one to accept faith as a viable tool in a new paradigm, and to act as a counterbalance to bureaucratic disenchantment.

Something conceptual and impalpable in this reified system can be helpful as an adjunct when things go wrong with one's health, and they always do. The cold steel of science and big business do possess a melting point, perhaps too high for some, too low for others.

Finally after a quarter century of teaching medical students, interns, and residents I learned that by making a topic fun, more is acquired. My irreverent and intermittent sportive style in no way should be construed as an attempt to make light of this grave disease. It is anything but.

This chapter will present a rather generalized seething indictment of organized religion and an apologist's defense of faith. They are not treated as 2 separate potholders but as 1 weaving cloth where the warp and weft are latticed. I did this because I think disparate ideas, especially those about a vast subject are best expressed in close proximity of each other. This suppliant author has tried to be fair with his counterpoise. If I have failed then once again let me apologize. In the end every individual gets to choose where on the continuum they ultimately lie.

That being stated I was totally secularized and agnostic for the majority of my time on earth. As alluded to on page XX when my daughter almost died I became unhinged and prayed daily at the hospital's chapel during her prolonged stay. Upon her recovery I had promised that I would never again label myself an atheist. I kept my word at being a coward. I have no regrets as she is a healthy and beautiful 31 year old. I am blessed. Even after the concatenation of draconian surgeries, which included the removal of my testicles, cancer, disability, profound hearing loss, and one pulmonary embolism I stood pat on my noncommittal ideology. But PRIOR to the embolism that almost killed me I began to open my mind up to the possibility of an elevated sanctity. Without that sea change in my thinking I would not have survived my PE and its aftermath mentally and ultimately physically. I also finally began to see and then realize from a bird's-eye- view as to why so many of my patients were allegiant to their religion.

I have no interest in having this penultimate chapter come across with that which is all too commonplace- which is a person befallen by a tragedy or undergoing a sudden crisis of consciousness becomes miraculously reborn into some religious doxology. Interesting but I don't think many would pass the intellectual sobriety test on this overcrowded turnpike. Today's breathalyzers are exquisitely calibrated.

There are many examples of this rather predictable phenomena. Saul of Tarsus (modern day Turkey) on the road to Damascus underwent an apoplectic/epileptic meltdown and was forever transformed. From a 21st century physician's lens this is not surprising as epileptics, if indeed he was, often report experiencing "visions" once they literally come to their senses. Depriving oxygen from the brain for a period of time will produce the same dizzying reports. Previous to the miraculous scratch on his cerebrum the Judaist Saul is portrayed as a rather angry fellow persecuting innocent Christians considering them perpetui inimici (enemies of life) and treating them with heavy-handed zeal. He eventually limned into the Apostle Paul evangelizing in the name of Jesus Christ throughout the Levant. He avoided Jerusalem for approximately the next 3 years as he became somewhat deracinated from the maelstrom of first century revolutionary politics and its powerbrokers in Palestine. The denizens of Jerusalem and its suburbs were still trying to cope with the Roman occupation and the myriad of "saviors" crucified on an almost daily basis along with the occasional OBE (out of body experience). Although only one made it through the final cut or so it is verily written.

If I may be permitted to digress it is my belief that the Jewish people at that time were manifesting some psychiatric disorders after centuries of losing control of their own destiny. This probably began around 721 BC when the Jews were conquered by the Assyrians. One hundred and thirty five years later, in 586 BC they were routed by the Babylonians and their iconic First Temple razed during the siege. Cyrus the Great of Persia, considered a messiah sent by G-d, *permitted* the Jews to return to Jerusalem in 539 BC. I kind of think that is how he obtained the messiah sobriquet. They would be subjugated by Alexander the Great less than 200 years later. The Hellenistic Period was a time of great assimilation and cultural identity theft. After Alexander's feverish demise (possibly typhoid or malaria) in 323 BC his generals divided up the imperium. The Hebrew state would be caught in the vortex between the Seleucid Empire whose capital was in today's Syria and the Ptolemaic political machine of Egypt featuring Cleopatra and her asp. The Israelites would become vassals of both until the Hasmonean Dynasty of 141 BC. The Roman general Pompey captured Jerusalem in 63 BC.

I would think by then the polytheist Jewish internal spiritual ideology was changing as rapidly as their travel gear. Certainly the prophets at the time seemed to be preaching along that crooked fault line or was it why-is-it our –fault line. Despite flurries of self- determination the Romans would be their new masters for approximately the next 400 years. The scholar and ex-cenobite Karen Armstrong posits that the "demons" Jesus and the others were purging (some magically transferred to the innocent swine) were in essence varied sick and agitated mental states. As a first generation American I saw first- hand the mental disordered demons caused by dislocation and upheaval in my agnate grandparents and father. When my dad at age 96 was in hospice and semi-comatose his final words in a repetitive and plangent voice were "I'm from Russia." He probably never fully left and that is only one human being one crop removed. I can only imagine the psyche of those inhabiting the first century with such collective internal and external Sturm und Drang. Is there any wonder why they were over-reaching for miracles and messiahs to get them back to Canaan? The land of milk and honey must have seemed a million miles away.

The curmudgeon Martin Luther prior to hammering his 95 theses in 1517 on the church door at Wittenberg which helped accelerate the Protestant revolution along with Guttenberg's new printing press evidently was hit by a lightning bolt in in 1505. This supernal sourced energy field converted him from potential lawyer to a monk with astraphobia, but he remained an inveterate bigot. His quote "The person of the Antichrist is at the same time the pope and the Turk" kind of says it all. The anti-Islam polemic was also spewed by the Catholic and Jewish theologians and Big Marty often appropriated theirs for his own needs. To be fair many of "enlightened" philosophers including our Founding Fathers and Hebrew polymath Moses Maimonides were also very critical of the "Turk" (Islam). The latter also appeared to be quite the racist judging from some of his written work. Dr. Luther initially cut the Israelites some slack but when they decided not to obsequiously follow, his axiomatic anti-Semitic ranting could not leap from his quill fast enough. He probably would have been a great attorney if not for the heavenly electrostatic charge. With the Reformation accelerating something had to replace papal authority. That replacement was the Bible and the unvarnished word of Yahweh, and so the world once again began to dramatically change.

With all his personal interstices Luther appeared to be a moral man and helped loosen the collar of Catholic dominance in Europe despite his tendency to point the rigid hortatory finger. I think most would be surprised to recognize his feeling that Church and State should be separate though Jesus's quote "rendering to Caesar" implies the same. Quite the enlightened opinion in the 16th century where paradox and kings were coregents advised by holy men. This despite his propensity to ignore the ineluctable yoke of reality. He saw the light as well as getting struck by it and like most, once you see it there is virtually no possibility of un-seeing it.

The lugubrious and hyper earnest Saint Francis of Assisi who seemingly conducted direct conversations with G-d was converted from an entitled bar-hopping dissolute war-like womanizer to one of the most respected and revered mendicant icons in Catholicism. I personally think he was as close to Jesus-like then anyone I have ever studied. However the virgin Saint Clare of Assisi and he may have shared more than the same birthplace. That stated when one reviews his nuclear family dynamics particularly the parental relationships, we see the need for a future psychiatrist. It would come to no surprise that the man who spoke to birds and self-flagellated for feeling cloy needed a mental health provider. Blessed be the straitjacket. The rest as they say is history, and history it has been stated is "one damn thing after another."

Quite frankly the list of "divine" interventions and conversions goes on and on and will be debated till the "End Days" of Revelation kicks into raptured gear. The canard of the magical *woo-woo* soul will hopefully be exposed when science proves that it stems from our own electrical impulse derived from chemical reactions. As neuroscience motions forward I hope that concept will one day materialize as the other simultaneously disintegrates. Hopefully there will be an evolution to the dogged primal abstraction.

The human brain is responsible for 20% of the energy used by the body despite being only 2% of the total body weight. Its primary fuel source is glucose (sugar). My sense is that some of the hidden extreme calorie expenditure is allocated to the numinous *soul*. In fact if a nerve cell (neuron) was connected to a pair of earbuds one could actually hear the output in the form of rhythmic clicking. When the brain dies, we die along with the clacking. The French philosopher and mathematician, Rene Descartes who defended the duality of the mind and body probably would not be happy with today's scientific findings. C'est la vie (It is life), until it isn't Monsieur.

Imagine if all the insubstantial stories were put to rest with that acknowledgement. In my view our quintessence does pass on to another unique world but I do not believe it to be a heavenly kingdom nor a devilish basement. I think our soul is passed on to our progeny via memories and genes producing atavistic traits. I often feel my grandparents and parents within me. "Okay I'll eat, hassle me not!" I think their final resting places are neither final nor resting.

Consciousness, spirituality, thoughts, and the entity we call the soul do seem linked but what happens when we are rendered unconscious. Does the spirit go to sleep? If so that puts a god into a very strange position during the news blackout. My reckoning is that the newfangled psychologist would have a field day with these fairy tales alongside the dogmatism and sclerosis that they have spawned. Every reverent book appears to be strewn with every personality disorder but it does not gainsay the fact that these three influential men despite their odd coiffures and countless other humans were inspired by something less than obvious and tangible. After all, grasping the intangible is a sign of intelligence and found in many a human endeavor. Prince, Sting, Bono, Jay-Z, and Madonna are extant examples and even some with last names like Einstein, Newton, Planck, Maxwell, and Hawking. Intangible however does not necessarily translate into divine or magical.

In my case as previously stated I was an atheist/agnostic since graduating from Pennsylvania State University. I would make an obtuse reference to my ancestors the Israelites circumnavigating the Sinai for the same time period of four decades but the archaeological evidence appears a bit exiguous. There is interestingly more historical evidence of captured Hebrews around 70 A.D. (after their revolt and temple destruction) being an integral part of the workforce that built the Roman Coliseum. In a recent paper put forth by one of Israel's premier archeologist, he lays out the case against any such uniform sojourn of the "600,000" Jews from the hegemony of Egypt. The lack of proportionality is in itself dazzling. Not one campsite or circumcised muffin-head remnant found. Just a farrago of imputation and innuendo. Can you dig it? In all probability it was story that was no doubt modified over the years before being codified onto dare I say stone by those promoting their innovative desert doctrines. I think it is safe to suggest that more Jews migrate to the eastern coast of Florida annually from the northeast corridor of the United States than those who took leave of the pyramids towards the Red Sea littoral. These interesting yet desultory and aimless stories with often mindless fermented distillations were ubiquitously common to all ancient people's narratives. They were no doubt originally put into play to help create a particular cohesive identity and ethos- religious geopolitical, social, economic etc. to help with the baleful aspects of dragging about on a flat surface under the scorching sun.

These cultural selfie shticks would eventually help the predominantly agrarian sodalities limn into their respective nation states centuries later. Ridley Scott's Hollywood movie "Exodus and Kings" was banned in the United Arab Emirates and Qatar due to "the intentional gross historical fallacies." The Islamic censors might have been on to something and who among us can stand "fictionalized" fiction anyway? Not to mention Batman (Welsh actor Christian Bale) portraying Moses? The original writers who began writing about that which could have possibly been, after undergoing numerous revisions by many midlevel and rather imaginative scribes metamorphosed into that which could not possibly be.

The obvious thaumaturgies, a father with an Eastern European variant of oppositional defiant disorder (ODD), and Freud's *Future of illusion* jettisoned me into the waiting arms of Baruch Spinoza, John Locke, Thomas Jefferson, and Bertrand Russell. Organized religion appeared as anything but and the concept of an *All Knowing* appeared to be a human construct. Did he make us in his image or did we make him in ours?

I had gotten very angry at the "Big Guy." How could one so omniscient portray oneself in such a juvenile if not bipolar narrative? Loving, sentient, and stable and then moments later insensitive, deliriously demonical, and one-sided. From a plenary group of multiple gods the monotheists have reduced the number to one with multiple personalities, each with its own mood disorder. The new ICD-10 code for which is F44.81. Quite frankly I do not think the polytheist would recognize the prestidigitation. What characteristics made one tribe better than another? Characteristics formatted and ultimately handed down by him. Why did it seem that those who professed the most piety possessed the most incandescent and simmering hypocrisy, vitriol, and violence inside them?

What made *The Almighty* suddenly appear to the ignorant and mostly illiterate narrative-seeking Semites of the Middle East while the more stable and advanced civilization of yellow China was ignored? What was it about the viridity of boscage that he avoided and the desert that indulged his fascination? Was not G-d peripatetic and equipped for any weather system? Not to mention the brown people of India, the black people of Africa, and the red people of the Americas. How about those children? Could they not have accepted an abstract god as easily? Why was his language so monochromatic? Even if anybody is dewy-eyed enough to swallow the fallacy that the earth is 6000 years old what was the *Supreme Architect* doing for the first 3000 years, video games? Radioactive testing puts the real age at 4.543 billion years + or- one percent. Nice math skills! "The Guardian of Israel neither sleeps nor slumbers." It seems however he does enjoy his naps. The deadening force of tradition can sometimes be assuaged if it is permitted to countenance the obverse.

What I found more egregiously insulting was the public relation firms that G-d hired in the years to follow after his coming out party? Psychotic popes, bellicose imams, corrupt rabbis, power-thirsty monarchs along with their distaff equivalents, power brokers and dubious prophets. They all shared the insane quest for wealth, puissance, and control in this world but bloviated about the next. One needs simply to look at the two-tiered manorial system of feudal Europe where there were men of wealth welded to power and detumescent men of neither. Esurient aristocratic venerability not only supported the unfairness but were in part architects of it, often suppling the bilious torrential close-captions. Totally opposite of the socialist and egalitarian message of Jesus.

Even if one wanted to allow for a few millennium of a learning curve how does the unstable amalgam of James Bakker and his beguiled wife Tammy Faye(fey would be a more apt description) get to the top of the PTL (Praise the Lord) club? This deceptively simple and fetid dyad with a suspicious wealth of celestial information was allowed to flourish while representing a providence as they fleeced the gullible flock out of millions. The ongoing sub-rosa malversation came to a screeching surcease after it was discovered that hush money was paid to the sooterkin, one Jessica Hahn regarding an inappropriate relationship with the epicene lothario. Patently Reverend Bakker was in her "holy" waters surrounded by a not so innocent thicket. Further investigation would prove beyond a reasonable doubt that this was merely the tip of a very disturbed iceberg. An iceberg whose concretions began in anything but chilled conditions thousands of years earlier.

Jimmy (I have sinned) Swaggart is another example of a pitiful charlatan claiming telegnosis during his sulfurous sermons on Sunday and impious conduct on the weekdays. Jerry Falwell, the captious Baptist minister and homophobe declared that the attacks of 9/11 were an opprobrium brought on by America's un-Christian mendacious behavior. He did sayeth this foolishness with crushing certainty while the World Trade Center was still collapsing. Yep that was the reason, much like when he published that the purple Teletubby named Tinky Winky (a character from the BBC children's television show) was a gay role model for children. As marijuana becomes more and more legal, as the Confederate flag begins to descend further and further down the flag poles of State Capitols, and same-sex marriage is now officially the law of the land one can only wonder what the founder of the inappropriately named "Liberty University" would have said.

At least Presidential Republican candidates Rick Santorum, and Bobby Jindal are still with us for colorful commentary and will have plenty of time to provide more particularly after their failed political hustings. They are currently polling at .2 and .4 percent respectively. Keep praying boys! The only thing funnier was fellow bigot Pat Robertson's run for President of the United States in 1988. Although Rabbi Daniel Lapin alleging that the Bible warned us of the attacks on September 11, 2001 really got robbed of the 1st place trophy. Must have been an anti-Semitic conspiracy? Perhaps he should have been more definitive on September 10th. #Trending Hashtag Schmuck! Pardon my capacity for skepticism but representative legitimacy seems to be an issue when it comes to all persuasions.

One does not have to travel outside of America to see this more clearly than with Joseph Smith, founder of the Latter-Day-Saints (largest Mormon sect). The con man from New York professedly found divine message-laden golden plates in his neighborhood of Crazy Ville. Unfortunately Joe did not keep nor pawn the written revelation of G-d but handed them off to the fulgent angel Moroni. These plates told the narrative that Native Americans were scions of the lost tribes of Israel who sailed to the New World around 600 BCE. A reawakened and reconstituted Jesus in 34 CE then visited America and shared his gospel with them. Needless to say the story continues to devolve from the group's propitious start including the founder running for President of the United States in 1844. Unlike the movie "Mr. Smith Goes to Washington" this mountebank Mr. Smith did not. He did go to an Illinois jail the same year for destroying the office of a local muckraker exposing the fraud. Present-day –saints, doubtful. Latter-Day-Saints hardly.

The incessant paronomasia and unintentional word mismatches one finds on the weekly religious billboards are equally entertaining. "Soul Food is Served Here" is not too bad but "A Loose Tongue Often Gets in a Tight Spot" should be disambiguated. The same can be said for "The Best Way to the Top is on Your Knees." The other day I drove by a Catholic church whose sign simply averred "Heaven is Real." Unless they were streaming the eponymous movie from Netflix for their congregation it is difficult to take the insouciant statement seriously. WWW. Snopes.com agrees. When heaven is the subject there are obviously no unarguable propositions.

Billy Graham the former Fuller Brush salesman in his autobiography avers "I outsold every other salesman in North Carolina." I cannot imagine how many souls he swept off their feet with his muscular oratory and at what price. He would have been a great huckster during the 1730s and 1740s religious revival known as the Great Awakening. This does not necessarily mean he is a degraded man of G-d. There does however appear to be a nexus between the adult need for emotional consolation, rigid upbringings, cultural lunacy, poor parental imagoes, and natural salesmanship. These somewhat tainted origins can eventually gird a multi-million dollar phalanx in faith's secondary derivative market. Conversations that are documented at the Nixon library reveal that the good reverend not only agreed but jointly owned the anti-Semitic ravings of our Quaker president.

His son Franklin in June of 2015 urged a boycott of Wells Fargo Bank due to their television add portraying a lesbian couple anticipating an adoption of a child and was allegedly pulling millions of pious dollars from the institution. Bully pulpit indeed used as a grudging final resort in a thuggish way. One gets the eerie impression that Billy and his son would have been great administrators in the Lodz ghetto, Poland 1942 whose lot was just following a psychopathic leader in Berlin. He did issue a half-baked public apology after the Nixon tapes became public, however he did not remember the remarks. What was he apologizing for then? Liar -liar pants on hell- fire!

Despite his personal crevasses he consistently appears on Gallop's list of most admired men and women. When a POTUS (President of the United States) gets into trouble he is the spiritual adviser of choice. One wonders his burning advice to President Clinton regarding the hazards of cigars in grand jury investigations. Whether a world leader full of sardonic hauteur or a selfless world follower it appears to me that many of the steadfast keep two sets of books, one for the weekdays and the other for the weekend.

Cotton Mather (Eminem is Mathers) the prolific Puritan colonial minister who helped lay the groundwork for the 1692 Salem witch trials would be proud of his mega-rich made-in- America progeny and their television broadcasts. Broadcasts that are rather distressing in their gaping bandwidth. To be fair to Cotton he was also way ahead of his time and intermittently forward-thinking. He encouraged the widespread administration of the small pox vaccine when many in the medical community didn't. He also changed his stance on Satan being the cause of mental illness when he himself came down with a case of the "blue devils." Where would mankind be without the soggy perimeter made of situational ethics? He denigrated the viridescent crescent of Islam and derogated Muslim philosopher Ibn Tufayl's tract on how human reason led ineluctably to the existence of a G-d. However he was impressed enough so to include the *Mahometan* in his own writings. Interestingly enough the enlightened philosopher John Locke himself was influenced by the same "heathen."

Too many people forget that when a destabilized Rome collapsed and the Dark Ages ensued it was the Arab that kept the information technologies and highways open. Unfortunately in the 13th century the Mongols laid waste to Islam and its Golden Age was forever gone. One can argue that despite sparks of brilliance, the Arab Cimmerian veil then descended and has not yet lifted. One noteworthy exception was Persian intellectual Nasr al-Din al Tusi whose book entitled *Memoir on Astronomy* would have a profound influence on the Catholic astronomer Copernicus and his heliocentric model of the universe. A model that enraged the Catholic Church, Martin Luther, and other Protestant reformers since it disagreed with Bible inerrancy. Many people are as evidence-proof now as they were 500 years ago despite the ease of keystroke verifiability.

These are but a few examples of intelligent yet rather imbalanced disgruntled religious visionaries that have been called upon to spread the "Word" but acted at times ½ ape and ½ Neanderthal possessing a scornful decency. In Doctor Mather's case being named after an ungracious shrub could not have helped.

The ancients did not behave much better as we romanticize our sanitized heroes and photo-shop their flaws. The uxorious King David every bit the libidinous player and a votary of toothsome women in general wasn't the Goliath he is often made out to be. He ordered a hit on the soldier Uriah the Hittite so he could marry his wife Bathsheba who was carrying the King's child. Evidently Mount Uriah in New Zealand is neither named for the cuckolded soldier, nor for his wife's sexual preference. Moses in Exodus ordered to have 3000 innocent men put to death. Both figures are often depicted in the Bible as Samson in the field and Solomon in council but it appears that they both at times acted as Philistines. Joshua's utter destruction of the Canaanites upon entering the Promised Land would land him today at The Hague to be tried for crimes against humanity. Like him on Facebook. Move over Slobodan Milosevic.

The Quran says that those who disbelieve will be exposed to fire and taste the torment. A Muslim's reflection on the tome is considered inessential and profane. As I do not ascribe to any religion I think a reflection on the Qur'an narrative regarding Muhammad's aeronautic adventures on a white steed between Mecca and Jerusalem and beyond is necessary due to its incredulity. It is written that around 621 a flying mammal known as Al-Buraq taxied about the prophet Muhammad between the two aforementioned consecrated sites. In Islam it is called "The Night Journey." Accompanied by the Angel Gabriel the threesome also booked a few flights to different venues where they met some of the earlier ethereal prophets like Adam, John, and Jesus. Supposedly the never aging Al-Buraq in prior years taxied about the patriarch Abraham around the Mediterranean depending with whom the spry guy wanted to sleep. Certainly if this was viewed as allegorical then the story holds a scintilla of merit but millions have no doubt that this tommyrot is fundamentally true. One wonders how many people have martyred themselves with this fantasy as the last simulacrum etched onto their brain prior to engaging a trigger mechanism. Inessential and profane is an apt description. And to think that the prototype for the limousine service known today as Uber was a 7th century invention. Peace be with you, perhaps, but the god-fearing tome is full of fantasy and decomposing prose often used as a "How To" manual for things that should never be.

Jesus is decently silent about the ills of slavery and the

post- ictal St. Paul affirmed it after regaining his senses. While it is true that the abolitionist campaign in our country was led by Christians, we need not be too generous in its implication as the most egregious acts against slaves were committed by the same group. What we hold as "gospel" is often rhapsodized and gerrymandered to fit nicely into our cerebral cortex which at its core is reptilian. When one reads the biblical and Quranic narratives about the natural world there is nothing earth shattering but for their myths. Just an edematous corpus with misdated prophesies so camouflaged to be presented as broadcasted breaking news. How about a sentence or two on the then future 1929 stock market crash?

King David and King Solomon are described as having fabulously wealthy empires but there is no mention of either in the historical discourse. I thought money talks? If there was putative beauty to their dominions it did not emerge from the chrysalis historically. Nor is there vestigial archaeological evidence.

Despite a long list of pagan historians writing at the time of Jesus there is no record outside of the Bible about his execution and resurgence. Could you imagine a history book written today without a mention of Mr. Putin, Saddam Hussein, George Washington, Gorbachev, or Mandela? The prophesies tell us that Israel will extend from the Red Sea to the Euphrates; (Exodus 23:25) The Babylonian King Nebuchadnezzar will destroy the city of Tyre; (Ezekiel 26:7) Egypt will become a barren wasteland; (Ezekiel 29:8) The Nile will dry up; (Ezekiel 30:12) The Egyptians will speak the language of Canaan; (Isaiah 19:18) The city of Damascus will be razed; (Isaiah 17) The city of Hazor will be inhabited only by jackals; (Jeremiah 49:33) Not, not, not, not, not, not, and wait for it- not!

If in the Bible and Quran there are a multiple of prophesies proven counterfactual along with galloping gossip and hearsay why attach weight to any of them simply because they are beyond attempts at being proven falsifiable? Imagine evolution given that free pass. Would you hire a plumber off Angie's list using the same ersatz thinking? If only CCTV (closed -circuit television) traffic monitoring was available during the Bronze Age.

It is quite obvious that the Jehovah of the Abrahamic faiths (I have chosen to stick primarily with the big 3 for simplicity only) has not shown himself to be consistently civil. In fact his footprints nor scribbled "G" is anywhere to be found yet alone notarized.

Exceptional claims require exceptional evidence especially when grasping at molecules of truth. Where be it? In fact if we are so high on an omnipotent agenda why is life so unfriendly, entangled, often ungenerous, shrewd, and stressful? Why is evolution so time consuming, painful, experimental, and immersed in serendipity? If a celestial being created us as distinct forms why does evolution scream to us otherwise? Even the Pope admits to evolution in a somewhat doleful tone as well as other religious leaders. I do not think they are necessarily happy about it though as the encirclement of crisis is at the same time tightening and expanding all around them.

In a counter-punch attempt to devalue evolution certain members of the crowd have propped up the concept of "irreducible complexity" to support an intelligent design platform. Basically it argues that if one removes a part from an organism and it stops functioning then it must be irreducibly complex defying that it evolved. This is regarded as brabble and no legitimate scientific society endorses intelligent design. Quite frankly this hypothesis should be permanently packed away in mothballs, but why stink up the naphthalene.

The original vision-impaired microbes and the multitude of people who to this day choose to affirm the senescent musings of purblind Iron Age script writers share the same genes. I would prefer to hang out with the bugs. After all they survived long before us and will continue to do so long after we are gone. There are 10 times more microbial cells that share our body (microbiota) than there are human cells. Bacteria hold dominion over us, not the reverse. Antibiotics are but a laughable diversion for them.

When legates John Adams and Thomas Jefferson met with their counterparts from Libya, they were told that the Barbary pirates attacking nascent United States shipping and holding American sailors as captives were justified by the Quran. An excuse that continues to this day whenever there is jihadist violence directed at the West. What is interesting and most would find incongruous is that more jihadist violence is chiefly directed at other Muslims. Over 200 years later Libyan Judo athletes "flipped" out when asked to train in the same facility with the Israeli team during the 2012 London Olympics. Is there any doubt that animosities repeat themselves?

The American diplomats and many others were outraged that white Christian sailors were held for ransom by dark Muslim pirates never giving a second thought that the slave trade imprisoned Muslims from Africa for generations. Mr. Jefferson was too precise a thinker not to see them as cognate issues. The future President of the United States was like most of us, somewhat dismayed on most days which sometimes clouds judgment.

Whatever we have achieved or accumulated in our lifetime eventually gets dispersed into vapor with only a small percentage making it into written history. Hypocrisy is hypocrisy and it universally appears to be handed down throughout the wilderness of the ages.

When physician Baruch Goldstein opened fire in Hebron in an incident known as the Cave of the Patriarchs massacre, 29 Muslims were killed and 125 injured on the Purim holiday in 1994. It was because the palliative influence of the Torah gave him permission. We need not discuss the abjured Hippocratic Oath nor Goldstein's contemptible psyche. To many he was a saint and a hero. Perhaps he was trying to get even for the Hebron Massacre 65 years earlier where close to 70 Jews, mostly students and teachers were killed by Arabs during the European receivership. A mandate that sadly lacked specificity, simplicity, and synchronicity. Many of the close to 500 survivors in 1994 were hidden by local Arab families. The fringe lunatic was killed on Purim by some of the viable remaining members. At his funeral a not so timorous Rabbi Perrin said that "One-million Arabs are not worth a Jewish fingernail." No doubt a strained statement declared for effect given the heated occasion.

Goldstein was a supporter of the Kach political party which was founded in 1973 by the right-wing Zionist Rabbi Meir Kahane who called for the emergency Jewish mass migration to Israel because of the potential for a "second holocaust" in America. No doubt Neiman-Marcus and a fair amount of hair salons would soon follow. I assume his math did not include the earlier holocausts in America against the Native American or Negro yet alone the Turkish holocaust of the Armenians years before World War I. Kahane who also founded the Jewish Defense League (JDL) felt that Israel should be under the small-minded and parochial Jewish law as codified by 12th century jurist Moses Maimonides. Under this ideology there would be no fluid nor cultural exchange between non-Jews and Jews. One can only wonder how the former would have been enforced as well as the penalty for conviction. Meir was mired so to speak in controversy most of his adulthood which included a domestic terrorism conviction in the United States for conspiring to make explosives. I cannot understand why his party could not win a single seat in the Knesset (Israeli parliament) with such an enlightened and adjusted leader at the helm.

In 1990 while giving a speech, the evocative Kahane was assassinated in midtown Manhattan by El Sayyid Nosair. The Muslim assassin was acquitted but three years later was convicted of murder because of his involvement in the 1993 World Trade Center bombing. The killer might have had links to Al Qaeda and Osama bin Laden. If realized at the time perhaps the Manhattan tragedy rooted in the divine acceptance of Allah could have been foiled eight years later.

One wonders what the *Ya-Ya Rabbi-Brotherhood* thought of Minister of Defense Ariel Sharon when Israel Defense Forces (IDF) joined up with the Phalange, a Christian right-wing party in Lebanon. The unusual toenadering between the 2 Canaanite sovereignties was due to a planned joint retaliatory military operation. An action that was responsible for the massacre of predominantly Palestinian and Lebanese Shiite refugees in the camps of Sabra and Shatila. The Mossad intelligence was later proven to be flawed as to the perpetrators of the assassination that initiated the alliance and subsequent bloodshed. The Kahan Commission in 1983 homologated Mr. Sharon's guilt and fruitful collaboration. Ariel and his blood-soaked fingernails, later trimmed and manicured would be Israel's 11th Prime Minister 18 years later.

Just in 2014 in July radical Israelis burnt to death a young Palestinian boy in response to the Hamas randomized projectiles emanating from Gaza. The same radical group that uses innocent people as human shields in a quest for seventh century desert-sharia-law purity. These acolytes might think that they will get"72 Virgins" in paradise, but I wonder if they have given any deliberation that perhaps 72 mother-in-laws arrive with the bombastic package. Insanity might be spelled differently in Hebrew than it is in Arabic but the meaning is identical. What a life of repose it would be for all of us if we lived under the combination of Maimonidean and Sharia law. One could only imagine the daily volume of visitors to Pornhub.com?

When reborn President George W. Bush and the neo-conservatives finally got their dream come true fiasco and invaded ancient Mesopotamia, the nation we call Iraq, it was Scripture and faith-based initiatives that underwrote the "Moral Crusade" against the "Axis of Evil." Revelations indeed! America was the new expansive Roman Empire every bit the vulgar bully who cared little about what the rest of the Hellenized world thought.

It seemed every decade or two her rivals and alliances switched places producing a foreign policy that defied reasoning and consistency. A draconian tax policy, financial impropriety, and an over-zealous treasury-draining bellicosity would soon in 2008 cost Americans 13 to 16 trillion dollars in wealth along with 9 million jobs and 5 million homes. Whenever an empire gets too big for its infrastructure, its bridges if you will, there is always a Carthage simmering with insurgency on both sides of that nation's firewall.

Seven years later another Evangelical, former Senator Ron Paul from Texas is warning us of yet another upcoming economic crisis along with civil unrest. The televised admonitions are run more frequently when the Dow Jones stock Index is having a profoundly bad day. Fear and panicked thinking are the underlying fuel sources for all this inciting rhetoric. To all appearances Jesus has a summer home near Dallas. G-d's country, Texas, known for its football fervor, gun ownership, religious underpinnings, and state sanctioned executions (#1 by far). In a recent 2015 survey ranking credit card debt by municipalities, of the top five American cities, three were in the Lone Star state. Ostensibly many Texans pay for their pigskin-loving, rifle toting, and Bible-thumping lifestyles with American Express. Don't leave home without it. I assume the State pays for the lethal injection nostrum with cold hard specie. They should have enough cash on hand after defunding Planned Parenthood. Yahoo, love them cowboys!

The political Christian Right and their need for dogma over data has its wooden legs and fingerprints all over this mess. I suspect that hard-working blue collar made-in-America Christians will yet again bear the brunt of the next financial meltdown. Imagine a world that contained defenders of secularism and pluralism with ½ the zeal and a printing press that could create money prn (as needed)?

A Dutch filmmaker murdered (Theodoor van Gogh) because of a movie he produced criticizing the treatment of women in Islam. Abortion centers torpedoed by un-practicing barbarous Christians. Gynecologists prescribing to patients Bible passages to relieve premenstrual syndrome. Thirty years of refills should do the trick. A fatwa issued by the Supreme Leader in Iran Ruhollah Khomeini calling for the death of author Salman Rushdie. The Taliban and Al Qaeda could not have thrived if not for the religious sinews of Saudi feudal landlords, remnants of the

Hashemite empire, vast oil fields, Western intervention, Pakistan's corrupt military, and general Muslim discontent. These theocratic fascisms accompanied by conflicting loyalties and many more immoral and uncivilized actions are underwritten by the murky world of impervious divine writ. There are those who tend to idolize and others who tend to anathematize. My hunch is that the reflective yet unattached mirrors of history may one day sort out all the intangibles. Don't count on it.

It is not a stretch, to make the case at least in part that Israel is practicing both colonialism and apartheid in the Occupied Territories of Palestine. This based partly on the hodge-podge of the McMahon-Hussein Correspondence, the Sykes-Picot Agreement, the doublespeak of the Balfour Declaration, and World War I propaganda. Added to the fire was the decline of the Ottoman Empire, burgeoning Zionism, growing labor movements, an international chess game primarily between the British and French, and of course Scripture. G-d only knows that the Quran and Bible are dare I say replete literally with testaments of sexual abuse and violence begetting more sexual abuse and violence. It is in this empire often stated that Islam resorts openly to censorship and torture. No doubt but Judaism and Christianity wrote the guidebook, an actuality often dismissed. It is available on Amazon.com. Caveat Emptor (Let the buyer beware).

In the beginning, G-d created the world in 604,800 seconds. What took him so long was he aerobically unfit after doing nothing for 4.5 billion years? Soon to follow is Genesis 22, a pre-owned not so- generous-sui generis Babylonian myth. *Yahweh* "talks" to the patriarch Abraham or was it more likely a schizophrenic hearing voices? In this disturbing conversation he is told to "Take your son, your only son, whom you love-Isaac-and go to the region of Moriah. Sacrifice him there as a burnt offering on a mountain I will show you." Once again an insane amount of claims require an insane amount of evidence! More eloquently said by the French mathematician Laplace: "The weight of the evidence should be proportioned to the strangeness of the facts." Picture today a father about to immolate his son as per an invisible deity's command. What is more probable, an apotheosis of this imagery for perpetuity, or a scene replete with S.W.A.T. followed by numerous administered prescription medicines, reporters, tweets, psychiatrists, social workers, and imprisonment? Not to mention the son in high moral dudgeon appearing incessantly on "The Dr. Phil Show" taking the very drugs his crazy father should have been on prior to him gathering the kindling, a Bronze Age dripless turkey baster, and lighter fluid. Were marshmallows available back then?

Recently I was listening to Dr. Richard Dawkins re-tell the story of Sodom and Gomorrah on You Tube which when completed he asked some members of the audience if they believed the biblical story. To summarize the ridiculously insane tale, The *Almighty* made his intentions known to destroy the two cities of Sodom and Gomorrah because the people were deemed evil. Three disguised angels showed up at Lot's tent, who happened to be the only righteous man left in the vicinity. The male neighbors heard about the visitors and went to his humble abode to gang rape the visitors. Evidently there was no football on TV. It seemed as though the citizens were both profoundly wicked and bored. Lot, being the good man that he was proffered up his virgin daughters as a not so venial substitute. Fortunately the nearby residents were incapacitated by blindness giving Lot and his family time to escape but are admonished not to look back, as the Lord intends to carpet-bomb the municipalities. G-d does tend to smoteth in rather large numbers. Lot's wife, who may have been named Edith, could not resist the temptation and his turned into a pillar of Morton's salt by the omnibenevolent *Deity*.

After the escape his young daughters hatched a scheme to have sexual intercourse with their aged father to perpetuate his seed since the other men are up in smoke/smote. In the space of 24 hours they got him liquored up and had coitus seriatim which resulted in the simultaneous birth of Lot's children and grandchildren, Moab and Ammon.

Aside from countenancing a Bill Cosby form of dating as well as incest, why didn't the righteous father offer himself up to be gang raped instead of his children? What teenage girls on the run worry about anything but the ensuing weekend yet alone the ensuing generations? I would think food, shelter, clothes, drinking water, comfortable sandals, and make-up would be a priority. Not to mention the combination of alcohol and old age does not make for great erections yet alone conceptions.

When Dr. Dawkins asked a fellow on the first row if

he believed this Stephen King phantasm word for word, the man hesitated but mumbled through the excessive saliva "yes." I felt bad for the guy because there appeared a subtle sense of embarrassment similar to when one empties one's Halloween bag for the last time despite having a driver's license for three years. When Dawkins repeatedly asked how he could believe such an insane story, his answer was without hesitation: He believes in Jesus Christ and so the magic wand is once again waved. The frangible logic statement/equation goes as follows. "The Son of G-d exists therefore everything in the Bible must be true since it prophesied his existence." A: Jesus exists. B: Everything in the Bible is true. C: The Bible predicted the existence of Jesus. A&C∴□B. The Messiah, incontrovertibly via Genealogy.com was (or is it is?) a descendant of Lot through King David's grandmother Ruth, who is descended from none other than the *ill-conceived* child/ grandchild and concept known as Moab. These odd "lot" sequences and layered stories are found in the irreproachable hardcover that makes the Jewish people the only rightful landowner of Israel and is the foundation for the incubus to follow in both biblical testaments and Quran?

Indeed it may be an impossibility to decouple political rule from theological belief and this where a huge part of the problem lies even in nations with "walls of separation." One needs only to watch in our enclave a Republican National Convention and one is struck by the underlying Christian principles and principals that suffuse the event and beware their wrath if you disagree with the dying gasps of their arguments. Would you want to be on Sarah Palin's bad side assuming you can detect the good one?

Recently in the summer of 2015 Kentucky county clerk Kim Davis was found in contempt of court for refusing to issue marriage licenses to same sex couples in defiance of a Supreme Court decision allowing gays to wed. Despite three divorces the Apostolic Christian's excuse was that G-d's definition of marriage does not include homosexuals. Hopefully she can sort out her beliefs in jail bee-hive hairdo and all while reading about Lot and his daughters as her illegitimate children visit.

Whatever an individual wants to conclude seems fair but when the godhead is bought packaged with all the insipid accouterments, problems emerge exponentially. Difficulties that are often disjointed assaults on civilization. When a United States Congressman stated that climate change is a hoax because *Divinity* promised Noah that the world would never be destroyed again then we are all affected. Certainly when Senator Jim Inhofe from Oklahoma showed up ignominiously on the United States Senate floor with a snowball in hand attempting to repudiate global warming it assuredly proves that he is affected and is in need of prescription medicine for it.

Do you really want an eschatologist in the oval office anywhere near the nuclear launch codes? We had a few. In this nation it is so often easy to be armed with guns and so often difficult to be armed by facts. The latter having some of its roots in the arid badlands of antiquity. The wall between Church and State has more than a few interstices.

The brilliant Supreme Court justice Scalia seems adept at finding them with Justice Roberts not far behind.

When Muslim leaders do not accept valuable vaccines from the "Infidel" and infectious diseases begins to spread we are all affected. When the Land of Zion, whose eyes do not coruscate as it once had mandates that the Palestinians have no right to ancient lands because of a sacred writings compiled when the earth was thought a flatbread and not a matzah ball we are all affected. The hinge event of expropriation is very un-god-like and anguishing often accompanied by extreme brutality and mind-numbing caprice. Theocracies with unfettered nuclear capability are a very large grenade ready to detonate. It goes on and on and on and somehow with all the created red blood cells left to soak the earth a degage and redoubtable G-d is purportedly present watching the brutal massacres, pain, and disease. This with his arms akimbo for at least a hundred-thousand years and that is a conservative estimate of the time our species have been traversing the earth out of coastal Africa.

Does the *Almighty* require so much agony and how can he remain so jejune? What of the distorted cries and grimacing faces? Is that why everyday children starve to death along with a dearth of clean water, antibiotics, food, shelter, clothes, vaccines, and mosquito nets?

Was Hurricane Katrina and its subsequent flooding in 2005 with its 1245 deaths and 108 billion dollars' worth of damage necessary? The most affected states Mississippi, Alabama, Louisiana, and Florida, were ranked in 2014 by their professed religiosity as numbers 1, 3, 5, and 26 respectively. Why does #50 Vermont remain so pristine year in and year out? Why is it that every "Act of G-d" is a bad one similar to a Macaulay Culkin performance? How about the quotidian torment that many animals experience. What is the compensatory usefulness of suffering which appears universally in just about all religions including Hinduism, Tao, and Buddhism? Interestingly Islam and Jainism the latter of which heavily influenced Gandhi, are somewhat detached from the conceptualization. The Jains however deem that starving oneself to death is permitted which I doubt is painless.

In the badinage and persiflage of the Old Testament and Quran the wizened prophet Job, due to some devilish-double-talk from the *gangsta* Satan is stripped of his 401k which was then primarily invested in livestock, slaves, and land. The inveigling continued and the *Absolute Being* allowed the murder of Job's 10 children as well as most of his servants for "good" measure. This done to drive home a point regarding the disturbed connection between suffering and justice. Why G-d continued to countenance Satan's scurrility is beyond me. The miserable man remained pious and is restored to a happy younger man, free of every last maculation along with a spanking new etiolated "Brady-Bunch" family. Whatever the mimesis in the end it all worked out for the previous boil-laden Job who lived to the ripe old age of 210. Social Security was not pleased.

However what of the little bagatelle J.J. (Job Junior)

also known as Agnor, and his 6 brothers and 3 sisters? They are described as overbearing, materialistic, obnoxious in spirit, annoying, gloomy, unhappy, over- educated, smug, thin-skinned, and bacchanalian. Thank G-d *He* doesn't often visit a college fraternity or go to an "Old Navy" store on a Saturday afternoon. Is that why they got jettisoned from the earth's surface and where art thou? One would have an easier time finding a needle in a haystack or a brunette on Fox News.

St. Augustine labeled Job's wife as the "devil's accomplice." The theologian John Calvin, another brilliant disgruntled visionary designated her "a diabolical fury." The French-Fried beignet would use the same idiom for others. So with those ravishing reviews why was Mrs. Job allowed to hang around? It would seem the wanton murders of the children and indentured attendants were rooted not in negligence but intent. It would not be G-d's last manslaughter indictment. More importantly what happened to the sheep? All the pain in the world is inconsistent with an all knowing, all powerful, and loving G-d no matter how theologians want to defend this egregious behavior.

Is logic and good manners on a vacation cruise and if so were they infected with a food-borne illness? If we are to live a sentient and virtuous life should we rely on the primordial ignorance of primates based on autocracy and fear and why is there such a war against pleasure? Does the clitoris resemble Satan? Is the organ engorged, contorted, and fiery red? Does it force men to act immorally? Does it often belong to a succubus dangling temptation from below? Okay, does the clitoris resemble Satan?

Should we rely on the callous instructions to mass produce a spray that is repellent to women? Why is freethought and curiosity a felony? It seems to me that in general dogma at best will mollify and more often than not, stultify. No particular creator model successfully predicts the results of the natural world's pulchritude no matter how one tries to rig the game. Evolution though with some gaps does without the cyclone of inaccuracy.

Without evolution the Creation Story sounds like a rope of insanity tethered to an anchor weighted down with fragile hopes. Without it mankind is reduced to slavery because of a "not-so-garden variety" conversation with a slithering marplot who must have posed scripted questions in an unscripted fashion. Thousands of years later mankind is still paying the transaction fee at usury rates. Did I forget to mention the magical apple orchard and the rib allograft surgery minus the anesthesia for the birth of the slatternly Eve? A woman bamboozled by a reptile forced to wear the mark of her son Cain despite not yet giving birth to the malefactor.

Should we be surprised that in all religions orthodox men have been inculcated to despise women which at the same time increases and adulterates their rapaciousness in an unorthodox way? I am not sure what soft-headed author wrote this nugatory piece but it is safe to assume that hallucinogenic mushrooms were in full bloom and conterminous. A troop that would help define a leitmotif for the future treatment of femininity which includes stoning, burning, drowning, and sexual molestation. The Garden of Eden along with its misogynist roots could have used an in-house literary critic and a rotary tiller. Like the original language of the Bible, it is all Greek to me.

Without scientific innovation we as a species are grounded in fantasy. Holy books should just not be in the "Religion" section of bookstores but also in "Fiction," "History," and "Self-Help."

There may indeed be more to evolutionary theory than random mutation and natural selection but intelligent design is not one of them. 99.9% of species ever created are now gone which is expected when there is nobody with at least half a brain is doing the designing. Unless the clumsy designer is purposely producing a product not to last, like Microsoft's Vista operating system, the Ford Edsel, or the USFL (United States Football League). Complex structures do evolve from simplicity, evidence of immortality simply does not exist. If it did escape artist Harry Houdini would have reappeared unshackled and yet we are the ones that remain handcuffed. A complex neural network carries out these activities. This in contradistinction to the magical mystery tour our bedizened virtuous lecturers would have us accept as they bedazzle us from the lectern.

Electrical stimulation of the cerebral cortex has induced religious experiences, near-death-experiences, and out- of- body experiences. Reported miracles in all our glorified books have left us no evidence except for anecdotal stories along with supposed ear and eyewitness testimony. Why then were the laws of physics conveniently held at bay but not now? Is thaumaturgy really needed to explain life in the 21st century? G-d apparently has gone fishing and that is probably a generous scenario.

St. Paul when attempting to assemble a case for resurrection said that "Whatever you sow in the ground," after an exposition, "has to die before it is given new life." The early writings of the Church Elders compared the sun with rebirth because "it is withdrawn from our eyes, as if dying and is revealed again, as it were, by rising again." If you do not mind a subtle smirk the "as if" and the "as it were" sound like subterfuge *as it is*. Will I be put back together *as I am now* or *as I was* then? I forgive you Fathers as you know not what you say, nor what you write down onto parchment.

As evolutionary biologist Richard Dawkins states the universe was made with "pitiless indifference." Religion was our first attempt at philosophy when humanity was in its neonatal period. It is in our toddler years profoundly anachronistic and long ago reached diminishing returns.

Preachers, rabbis, imams etc. tell us that universal moral standards emanate from one figure and the writings he inspired but the data shows otherwise. Humans from all cultures, religions, cults, and non-religions agree on a common set of standards. Anthropologist Solomon Asch has said that "We do not know of societies in which bravery is despised and cowardice held up in honor, in which generosity is considered a vice and ingratitude a virtue." Birds have dangled worms from their beaks to feed fish. Dogs have nurtured and fed orphaned rabbits, kittens, and squirrels. Cats have done the same with puppies. Arabian babblers like other small birds warn others of trouble and donate food to each other. The animal world is brimming with right-minded actions.

In the Peter Freuchen's *Book of the Eskimos,* the author tells how one day after returning from an unsuccessful walrus-hunting expedition, he found one of the successful hunters from Greenland dropping off several hundred pounds of meat for him. After thanking him profusely the man objected indignantly: "Up in our country we are human!" said the hunter. "And since we are human we help each other. We don't like to hear anybody say thanks for that. What I get today you may get tomorrow. Up here we say that by gifts one makes slaves and by whips one makes dogs." Similar statements are found in the anthropological literature on other egalitarian hunting societies. I am pretty sure this philosophy came into being without a holy man or celestial dictator working his mojo through a church, synagogue, or mosque.

Who amongst us who is intact would not react to a child walking too close to the river's edge or into traffic? I have two children who have never formally set foot into any holy place except for the occasional bar/bat mitzvah, wedding, or funeral and they have never to my knowledge acted unethically. Their free-thinking secularized mother has a lot to do with that.

It seems that mammalian decency is instinctive and is modulated early on by good human connections made possible by the genetic wiring of evolutionary circuitry. These altruistic genes seem to exist because of hypothesized reasons such as genetic kinship, reciprocation as exemplified in the aforementioned exchange between the Inuit and the author, and acquiring a reputation for generosity. Israeli zoologist Amotz Zahavi has posited that altruism is an advertisement for superiority and dominance. Geneticists studying Y-chromosome data have found that nearly 8% of men living in the region of the former Mongol empire carry DNA nearly identical to the 13th century conqueror Genghis Khan. That translates into .5% of the world's male population, or 16 million descendants. Evidently his superiority and dominance not only allowed him to rule over the largest empire but helped populate it! Superspy James Bond (007) after 25 movies possessing the same traits may be a close 2nd. Unlike his martinis, the double agent's romantic interests were both shaken and stirred.

Thomas Aquinas and ensuing theologians have written that since humans have a moral conscience then G-d exists. The syllogism is totally lost on me. If that is true we would see better behavior in the devout. This simply isn't so. In fact a case can be made for the exact opposite. Noble prize winner Steven Weinberg wrote "That with or without religion, good people can behave well and bad people can do evil; but for good people to do evil-that takes religion."

The Pew Research Center reported in 2011 that the United States penitentiaries are bustling with religious activity. Not surprising in a jurisprudence system where prudence is rarely in excess. More than 73% of state prison chaplains say that efforts of inmates to convert other inmates are either common (31%) or somewhat common (43%). About three-quarters of the chaplains say that a lot (26%) or some (51%) religious switching among inmates occur particularly involving Muslims and Protestants. Also reported by a sizable minority of chaplains is that religious extremism is either very common (12%) or somewhat common (29%). The fanaticism is especially common among Muslim inmates.

So it seems that the fish tank known as the American penal system is teeming with schools of the god-fearing tepid as it may be, and not the godless. The Darwin-fish tattoo is no doubt a rare species in this social aquarium.

This is not surprising as religion has had a long history of authoritarianism and dispensing fear when dealing with freedom and justice for all. The supernumerary confection known as the Ten Commandments is interesting and worth a buried compliment or two, but is paltry and conflating next to the Code of Hammurabi and the genius of Athens in the 5th century before Christ.

Charity the often vaunted defense of the G-d fearing cannot be measured in a vacuum and is often uncharitable. The Shi'a militant organization known as Hezbollah is involved in many eleemosynary functions but is best recognized for its terrorist activities. The Catholic Church has a huge charitable arm but like other bureaucracies there are often unctuous hands dangling distally while scooping up the pelf. The Jewish charities were instrumental in getting displaced refugees in the 1940s out of Europe however the way they manhandled their friend President Harry Truman made him absolutely choleric. It is amazing that he did not leave office an imperishable anti-Semite. His personal diary revealed a waning warmth in his correspondences regarding the" Jewish problem."

My supposition is that religion's collective palms will remain more supinated in the future while intermittently and incorrectly predicting the exact day that this planet devolves into a conflagrant heap. Like their predecessors (in particular the Christian millenarians and the Jewish mystics of the "magical-last year" 1666) when the next year follows, it will be blamed on a convenient miscalculation. Blessed is the incautious calculator in the hands of those drowning in endless servitude. One wonders what the bedeviling headlines of The New York Times were in the year 666. Three digits by the way that will never be the first three on our Social Security cards as mandated by the United States Congress in 1935 due to its biblical association with the devil.

Not to be outdone by the federal government, Arizona and New Mexico officials had U.S. Route 666 changed to U.S. Route 491 because there was a belief that the road was cursed. Interestingly the Arizona State University Sun Devils play their home football games in Sun Devil stadium. The same state that does not allow their car owners to even purchase a vanity license plate with the number "666" on it. Unsportsmanlike and hypocritical conduct, 15 yard penalty!

Religions influence on economic development is also

worth a mention. One needs only to compare the life-cycles of North America vs South America. In the former the early settlers were primarily from northwest Europe where the Protestant Reformation along with its eponymous work ethic had the majority of its converts. Because of English law which included the Magna Carta (a document annulled by Pope-<u>not-so</u> Innocent III), parliamentary procedures, property rights, and individual civil liberties the immigrant's DNA was primed with somewhat open-minded constitutional principles.

This was not the same in South America. The indigenous inhabitants were forcibly Christianized and colonized primarily under the banners of Spanish and Portuguese Catholic absolutism and dogma. The infallible Church was the predominant influence and landowner by proxy. I think what is often lost with Columbus "discovering America" was that one of his prime motivations for navigation was religion. He was trying to find a route to India that would allow Catholic forces to outflank the Ottomans so Jerusalem could be returned to Christendom. I think we are lucky that the millenarian sea captain did not have a GPS.

Protestantism, hard work, the Enlightenment, self-reliance, free trade, republicanism, industrialization, technology, and capitalism would rise to new heights in the upper latitudes. What may surprise Donald Trump and others was that during intervals of heavy immigration to America there was generally and eventually correlations with periods of strong economic development. Nevertheless anti-Catholic sentiment, racism, and xenophobia were also unfortunately alive and well on the "welcoming" docks of America. South America has yet to comparatively emerge from the muck 500 years later. It appears to me that nation states with the most extreme ecclesiastic privilege have the least extreme democracies.

Most of 18th century Europe was gravitating to enlightened principles, centralization, secularization, and peacetime colonial trade to help in part firm up their balance sheets as the next century approached. The Muslim world shaken by the Ottoman disintegration especially after losing the 1683 Battle of Vienna, blamed the reverses on religious heresies. The Arabian Peninsula would come under the influence of preacher Muhammad ibn Abdul Wahhab who called for more Islam and less modernization and technology. The Europeans were looking forwards as the Arabs simultaneously were looking backwards and becoming radicalized. The once great empire deliquesced from Europe never to return. Their political decision to side with Germany in World War I was yet another nail in the coffin.

Did Wahhabism melt away with waning Arab world power and decreases in the standard of living? No it is the ultraconservative state-sponsored Sunni religion of 21st century Saudi Arabia. It is a source of global terrorism and the inspiration for the Islamic State of Iraq and the Levant (ISIL). Without petrol dollars the area would be as bankrupt as their fanaticism.

In the late 2000s Europe experienced a sovereign-debt

crisis which basically is the inability to repay or refinance public debt. The main culprits were the economies of Portugal, Italy, Ireland, Greece, and Spain. The derogatory anagram PIIGS was frequently used for the predominantly practicing Catholic and Eastern Orthodox nations (Greece). The Latin American debt crisis of the 1980s would throw Catholic South America into an economic tailspin for a decade. Coincidence maybe but recent data suggests that countries with higher GDPs are less religious and those with lower GDPs are more. America the beautiful is one of the outliers.

The previous paragraphs are just scratching the surface of a condition that needs a wide excision. That stated I also realized that there must be some good to all of this. I began to wonder in my 58th year why everyone from Abraham to Zachariah was responsible for reporting G-d's behavior any more than he was for defining theirs's and why should I believe them. Maybe G-d had been grossly mischaracterized and continues to be? So many people in the world are incessantly bowing down, gazing up, looking east, or facing west coupled to a primary number. Could they all be wrong or hoodwinked? Perhaps not everything in this world is made to make logical sense and sate the appetite of modernist analytical rigor.

I spoke to my spine orthopedist about this rather heavy luggage and he referred me to his priest for a good old sit down. I remember driving to the rectory and wondering what have I gotten myself into. Was this going to be any different from the other debates I have had with

Vatican ventriloquists? Was I in substance going to ask an Alzheimer's patient if he could recall possessing a good memory when he was in high school? In so much that the questions I had could not be easily unraveled and the answers forthcoming would be rambling, incoherent, and steeped in fantasy. I could not have been more wrong. It was a great hour and honor as we got along without effort.

When I brought up the usual cast of characters such as the Crusades, the Inquisition, the support of the Nazi regime, and anti-Semitism, he made no excuses. When I raised points about the promotion of racism, sexual repression, the treatment of women, homophobia, and the church's record of attempting to thwart scientific advancement he produced no alibi. When I inquired as to why Slovakia a rather nascent outfit run by a "good" Catholic regime during WWII was the most zealous in exporting the Jews east to the oven pits of Hell he appeared genuinely hurt. I dared not inquire as to why there was not one Catholic Nazi ever excommunicated by the Pope or what was his view on Catholic complicity with the twin killing machines of the peninsular Roman government and Italian fascism. When I asked him what value lies in a hallowed book that bolsters the argument of both the slave holder and abolitionist, he simply brought up the interpretation card. A card I generically find artless but his mellifluous presentation was apologetically sincere.

When I restated and at the same time mangled the French philosopher Diderot's aphorism that the world would be better off if the last king was hung by the entrails of last priest, he smiled as to say that the quote had some merit. Actually it is "Men will never be free until the last king is hung with the entrails of the last priest." I am sorry Denis. When I posited the conjecture that the very early Jewish commonwealths were torn asunder by influence peddling priests, he looked a bit askance. When I asked why Catholic doctrine is at the same time captivated by and yet infringed upon by the "holy" vagina he blushed. At least three times he apologized for his religion's sins and never did I feel the tension of opposing forces. The good man spoke of faith, hope, salvation, and forgiveness.

I was interested about what the good Father thought warts and all, but was more interested as to how he thought. I came in as a graceless taut bow and left as a grateful loose taught lyre. I realized that by focusing on religion's vices and ignoring its reforms was a cardinal sin. I was struck by the realization that by not formerly recognizing some truth in the past, I was obligated to be more open to different ideas in the future. He, like Dr. Kelly at Abington hospital was a good man doing a good job for what I was beginning to realize may be a good G-d.

Previously to leaving he placed his hands on my head and blessed me. I went to the icon laden church across from his office and sat alone to process the whole thing sitting back to behold the spectacle. I was not hit with a bolt of lightning, infused with magic juice, or motivated to genuflect to any sacerdotal imprimatur. I did gain some insight that day much in conflict with my tenaciously held worldview. Even the gray-haired fool evolves.

I was by no means buying any dogma hook line and sinker but I was willing to follow the lure cautiously via the serpiginous route. I was beginning to wonder that though in my view religion was initially breastfed lacking in nutrients did that necessarily mean it was currently malnourished. I think death probably lasts for a while. After all the mutilating surgeries I began to question was there a reason for it all that defied reason and did faith have at least a modicum of wattage that could be illuminating?

Three weeks after our palaver I experienced the pulmonary embolism that shattered me and continues to do so to this day. I amused myself that perhaps the righteous man used some Latin catachresis during his beatitude or made the sign of the Cross backwards. In my heart I knew it was an unfortunate random scientific event. Perhaps it was time to search for more vacuity inside myself and begin to pay attention to unimpeachable sounds of my neurologically mediate inner voice.

I started to think back on all the books I had read authored by the non-believers. I was drawn intellectually to their brilliant elocutions (most of them imbedded in this chapter) and luminous expositions such as multiple galaxies, quantum theory, Planck time, and how simple chemicals if exposed to the right conditions can morph into something called *life*. I was not wholly won over even then and somewhat turned off by their haughty expressions and their swollen egos that accompanied their great brainpower. The new atheists it seemed implied that believers are stupid, naïve, and half-witted. Nothing could be further from the truth. Some of the smartest and most educated people I know are devout believers from all sects.

To get a feel for their intellectual godless armamentarium one needs only to peruse the physics book entitled "Schrodinger's Cat" which involves a thought experiment involving a rather unlucky feline in a box replete with poison and a radioactive source. At the end of this short Disney flick we are left with the unflinching conclusion that the four-legged whiskered grimalkin is both simultaneously alive and dead. This in some way attempts to explain the dual nature of light which supposedly can exist as both wave and particle. Nevertheless the fluorescence and lucidity are lost on me and no doubt confuses the ailurophile and ostensibly everyone else

The physics community have now come up with the sub-atomic bosom, sometimes referred to the god-particle which has helped shed light on the Big Bang. A mere micro- second after a mysterious energy field exploded and every object we now know was created, after things cooled down a bit of course.

A very common argument that I hear and have often used myself as I did with the good Father was how religion is responsible for the Crusades, the historical carnage in Europe, continued genocides, etc. I think a little discussion on war is necessary as closer inspection is required.

I am pretty sure that WWI, WWII, the wars in Korea and Vietnam would have been fought if there was not any religion or just one worldwide religion. There is never one cause for war (casus belli) and though there are religious underpinnings to a fair amount of history's battles one cannot discount the ideological, economic, political, social, financial, and historical reasons. Some of these reasons have produced strange bed partners. King Francis I of France made a 16th century alliance with the Turks against his fellow Catholics, the Habsburg Empire. French Cardinal Richelieu supported the Protestant princes against the same coreligionist dynastic congeries a century later. The most significant ruler of the Muslim world Suleiman the Magnificent poured a ton of money into Protestant countries to keep Catholic Europe destabilized to help with his own conquests and defensive strategies.

We revisit the anti-religion argument again and realize that no matter the side, faith has done little to stop past feuds and has been anything but an emollient. It has yet to tip its hand indicating that a reversal is upon us. Will the subtext always be "My god's biceps are bigger than your god's biceps?" Will faith continue to provide the fossil fuel for human rights violations, misogynies, chauvinism, xenophobia, and terrorism? History is replete with religious internecine strife and it is impossible to absolve religion completely for man's bloody battles. It may not have created the bomb in a vacuum but has often provided the match and shortened fuse. Anything highlighting an "us" and a "them" ends ultimately in toxicity. One needs only to gaze at the current intra-Muslim Shia-Sunni violence. The cost of maintaining a world consisting of the victor and the vanquished is prohibitive and incoherent. Iraq and Afghanistan continue to be evidence of war torn disasters.

To borrow a phrase from President Woodrow Wilson, can there ever be "Peace without victory?" To me victory without peace appears to be the norm. Wars breakout, peace oozes reluctantly especially when religious factions are involved. Interestingly believers tend to point the minatory finger at the violent atheism of communism and the wars it has generated but that political theory was not born out of disbelief. Besides it later became evident that Stalin and the Russian Orthodox Church were quite cozy during WWII. Decidedly byzantine. The same church that kept slavery alive in the form of serfdom.

Certainly the recent hostilities in the Balkans, the Middle East, East Timor, Nigeria, Bali, Sudan, Sri Lanka, Indonesia, Beirut, Mali, Great Britain, France, Spain, Darfur, and Somalia seem to have religion's blessing littered all over their respective nihilistic bloodied battlefields. Just in November 2015, 71 years after the Allied liberation of Paris "The City of Lights" was again set aflame due to the coordinated and incoherent jihadist attacks by the Islamic State (ISIL). This organization will not waver from the indefatigable precepts embedded in Islam by the Prophet Muhammad. They have called on Muslims in the Western countries to find an infidel and "smash his head with a rock," poison him, run him over with a car, or "destroy his crops." Their commitment to reincarnating 7th century jurisprudence and ultimately bringing about the apocalypse is nothing but psychotic. The 1944 best- selling book *Is Paris Burning?* by Larry Collins and Dominique Lapierre will no doubt pullulate a sequel with the same title. History indeed repeats itself often with a different cast of actors. If one was to equate war with a house fire the ensuing arson investigation would often find evidence amongst the ashes that religion acted not as a flame retardant but as an accelerant.

That stated let us give some believers some due. Foreign policy and mind-rotting greed do not always bow down to a specific deity or cult. Many of the faithful were and continue to be appalled at what has transpired. There is often a lack of collateral, hard currency, and courage to change the historical vector. Religion has a slew of problems but the default scapegoat should not be painted with wide strokes.

Even though Pope Urban called for the 1st Holy War at the end of the 11th century, there were a multitude of reasons other than trying to recapture Jerusalem and destroying the infidels. One of which was to keep young trammeled men with their patrimony pending off the borders of monarchs with whom he was a signatory. Urban recognized that penurious young men with increased quantities of testosterone and swords could pose a problem. In other words what does one do when there is nothing to do? Make up something. This Pope and many of his colleagues were used to fishing in troubled waters.

Many of the non-believers also possess an unbelievable grasp of philosophy, history, game theory, rhetoric, diction, and mathematical logic which seemingly allows them to disarm and dismantle arguments of faith in a facile manner. This is done with some fascinating word-play but there does appear to coexist some incomprehensible beguilement. Conceivably the legerdemain is embedded in every pun and paradox.

I remember as a busy physician not finding the time to visit my parents. When my mother was diagnosed with dementia, she began to lose weight and steadily was withering away. As the disease progressed I began to see *more and more of her*, only to simultaneously *see less and less of her*. She expired in 2001. I have yet to forgive myself for the nonsensical treatment. She deserved better. I should have seen more of her when there was more of her to see. I would not make the same mistake with my father.

Take the "Barber's Paradox" vaguely attributed to philosopher and mathematician Bertrand Russell. It goes like this: There is a town with one male barber. In this town, every man keeps himself clean-shaven. He does so by doing one of two things: He either shaves himself or goes to the barber. Another way to state this is that "The barber is a man in town that shaves only those who do not shave themselves."

The question then is who shaves the barber? He can either shave himself or go to the barber (which is himself). Either way this results in the barber shaving himself, but he can't because he can *only shave those who do not shave themselves.*

Now take that reasoning away from a very real tonsure to a very abstract deity with suspect origins and one is left with the famous Abbott and Costello tautology "Who's on first? Is death a *viable* option? All this clever phrasing perhaps is interesting but the gravamen if there is one is often camouflaged within the piquancy.

Though I think scientists can often be very hard on and degrading to believers, these connoisseurs of inquiry should be the last collection of people ignored. We once again flip the coin in favor of the secularists. They bring up the most magnificent points and ideas and is the group, particularly the physicists most associated with under-standing the workings of the awe-inspiring universe. Not to mention making our daily lives infinitely more comfort-able and overall better. When Albert Einstein predicted that a clock runs slower in a gravitational field as observed by someone outside that field, most people then and now could care less. This phenomenon is called gravitational time dilation and is derived from theory of general rela-tivity. However what people would care about is that if our GPS did not correct for gravitational time dilation we would not always wind up where we wanted to go. Imagine the computerized sexy voice saying "You have arrived at your destination-I think?" All our electronic gadgets whether they be tablets, cell phones, comput-ers, electronic tracking devices, watches, etc. have a little piece of Archimedes, Newton, Euclid, and others embed-ded within the microchips. Where would we be without these people, deranged and fruity as they might have been along with their collective prickling of ambition?

I was amazed to learn after reading Dr. Victor Stenger's *God: The Failed Hypothesis* that our sun only allocates 2 photons out of a billion to warm earth, a planet found in the backwater of the universe where the majority of the mass isn't. Imagine an engineer making a heater that inefficient with a meager amount of parts readily available? Intelligent design? Hardly. Why is there "something" instead of "nothing"? Dr. Lawrence Krauss explains in *The Universe from Nothing* that "Nothing" is inherently unstable. It has been said that it takes "fine-tuning" to make the building block carbon hitherto only the *Prime Mover* could have fine- tuned the cosmos.

Interestingly experiments have proven that complex molecules based on carbon can be produced by simple substances. I recently read that only .0002 of the mass of the universe is the all-important carbon which is needed for human existence. Why did G-d give us so much helium and so little carbon? Was he contemplating a burgeoning balloon industry? A greater supply of lithium would have been nice considering anticipatory battery usage. Why would he send his only son to an agonizing death to redeem an insignificant amount of carbon posits the aforementioned scientist Stenger?

However throw in enough arcane complex theories, confusing ambivalences, the infinity concept, word games, and numbers followed by a plethora of zeroes and anything is possible as to the origins of man and the cosmos. It seems that for those who believe in a deity or those who believe in the dead-live cat, or is it the live-dead cat require a *quantum* leap of faith. Maybe faith simultaneously does all that it is purported to do for some and nothing for others? An *Almighty* that transcends time and space sounds very much like that energized microsecond prior to the Big Bang. Francis of Assisi, a Hindu Mystic, and Stephen Hawking seem to share the same divine vision, at least in part. The aforementioned Jainism rejects the scheme of a creator and postulates a universe eternal with no definitive beginning or ending. This Jain concept in some ways resembles a theory in physics known as *quantum tunneling*. This theory suggests a macrocosm that is due to collapse but can actually tunnel to the "other side" and emerge as a new expanding universe. That hypothesis sounds like it could be contained in The Apostle's Creed. Heisenberg Uncertainty indeed avers the poet.

It may be a lethal heresy to suggest that the leap is one in the same but perhaps both groups consider some god but disagree as to its nature. In the end it appears to me that it is impossible to lay down a general formula for it all. Unless vacant it will be purely partial in operation and that attempting to replace the chaos with a clearer view will forever be no easy task. If there is indeed a code it may be utterly undecipherable despite the underground Large Hadron Collider (LHC) beneath the French-Swiss border near Geneva. This is where brilliant particle physicists are attempting to prove what some theoretical scientists have suggested.

The practicing Jew, Muslim, Christian, or Atheist (and they should continue to do so) would look askance and sneeringly at someone practicing omphaloskepsis (meditating while gazing at one's belly-button) at least in the West. That being averred with 9 billion or so DNA pairs in the human genome I began to wonder if G-d was not ensconced in one or more of those sequences. If he can exist in the Trinity, why can't he exist in the infinite world of nothingness or molecular possibility? G-d may be residing in us symbiotically as a backdrop in our collective sub- consciousness and not actuating on anything. What we have interpreted as something that is heavenly directionalized may be nothing but nature's entropy. Is the inward looking navel dwelling humanoid from the East as directionally challenged as he or she is assumed to be? After all when it comes to Jehovah's residence there seems to be a lack of historical witness and ubieties.

It sounds a bit crazy but so does banging ones head against a rather weather resistant Western Wall, wrapping oneself up in black Tefillin, eating a divine wafer followed by a "Holy Water" chaser, or wearing an outfit with only eyes exposed covering up the beauty of G-d's creation. All in the arcana of finding the *First Cause* not to mention the untidy tax-free business of it all.

Eliminate all the irksome spokesmen, the propaganda and the draconian not-at-all petty manipulations that have laid waste in the name of Lord, and at the core there exists I think a more evolved version of a deity. The waning pulse of his biographers, the tangential camarilla and their abusive crowdfunding is not necessary. Man-made rules stemming from the wanton musing of predominantly narrow-minded men in their consistories along with theoretical dogmatizing is at best specious and at worst dangerous. A G-d that appears to be more user friendly is individualized and somewhat compartmentalized, and not one that is monopolized, capitalized, aggrandized, and ultimately politicized. A little less unscrupulous behavior would be nice. There might very well be a moral or two in the stories of Lot, Eve, Joshua, Mohammed, Moses, Jesus, and Job but they are entombed in the sarcophagus with so much that is immoral. G-d.2 may be a better operating system when the miracles written by imaginative humans are stripped away.

Whether G-d is linked to the pre-figuration of a glamorous celestial state where rewards and punishments are handed down I do not know, nor does the splendidly robed religious leader. One has the option at best to implicitly intuit the possibility but to take the position that it is or is not a "sure bet" is in my view arrogant and ludicrous. Maybe the *All Knowing* is a non- linear process or just the actual "thought" that he exists where there are no defined coordinates?

I love Big Bang, String Theory, Evolution, and Quantum, but even over millions upon millions of years I do not think it can explain the infinite complexity and profundity of one living cell yet alone the workings of the trillions in a human embodiment. 3.72×10 followed by thirteen zeroes to be inexact.

I use the word "think," and here yet again climbs the rollercoaster, because there is growing data showing that complex material systems do exhibit a natural process called self-organization which appears in living and non-living systems. The Fibonacci sequence (where the next number is found by adding the 2 previous-0, 1, 1, 2, 3, 5...) as an example is found repetitively in everything from stock market analysis to nature itself, such as flower growth. This somewhat imperils a design argument. In another words simplicity can limn into complexity, no architect is needed. The delicate balance between fibrin formation and fibrin dissolution is astounding in itself but is that due to a supernal engineer, partially perhaps? The human protoplasm if designed could have been mass produced better, but it only has to last long enough to reproduce and raise its young. Most of the time this is precisely what occurs. The real mediocrity in the "design" is often not exposed until after our reproductive capacity. I would have preferred a better warranty if not for the labor, then the parts.

Are we not a bit arrogant when we anthropomorphize him as we do our smart phones? Are we not a bit dovelike when we accept that which is preached from an elevated dais regarding a jeweled firmament, a long flowing white beard and toga, circulating angels, and a Burger King Diadem resembling those worn at the neighborhood's Renaissance Faire? One would think there exists a heavenly Maiden Lilith responsible for the choreography prior to the big art shoot?

In physics the Heisenberg Uncertainty Principle conveys that we can only know the statistical distribution of atomic particles in regards to location. In other words we do not know their exact location at any exact point in time. The concept of exactness is intrinsically imprecise. Maybe with the *Creator* we do not know and cannot possibly ever know at any given point *where* he is or for that matter *what* he is. Perhaps he is at times immanent and at other times transcendent. Would that not be enough? With all the theories there has to be in my head at least the possibility of an *Uncaused Cause* but I do not postulate it to be a probability attaining the standard of beyond reasonable doubt. Beyond unreasonable doubt perhaps and what is so immoral about that? The universe is so made that no one explanation makes total sense to me as to its origin. There are indeed perforations.

I am reasonably sure that after Charles Darwin returned from the most important cruise in history (no disrespect to Noah or Columbus) and would have been asked upon decamping the HMS Beagle if there was a G-d, he would have answered in the affirmative. To many the Englishman created a world upside-down but was it in reality made right-side up? There are those who think that one cannot love any deity and Darwin. They should open their minds as did the gentleman who forged the road to understanding nature's sublimity and who would forever banish the immutability of species.

We see revered men and women ululating particularly on the weekends with such false authority and self-righteousness that I cringe. They bear a striking verisimilitude to the wide-eyed lunatic at the racetrack screaming psychotically at the horse he wagered on because in the last race the animal finished a distant 5th. Worse yet he expects the horse to respond to the verbal philippic. Where is

Luther's lightning bolt when needed? There are some moments in time that I think the *Uncaused* is itself nature or was that bundle of energy that exploded in one microsecond second.

Mankind's incessant anthropomorphizing is in itself blasphemous and quite frankly intellectually incoherent. There is a whole industry that makes a fortune claiming that which they cannot begin to understand yet alone know.

These cringing moments often direct me back to my childhood. When I was six I remember quite vividly when my "first girlfriend" then 5, told me that I was going to burn in Hell because I did not believe in Jesus Christ and my tribe killed him. I immediately became terrified running home to my parents in tears. Rarely were they ever on the same page but this time they were. My mother and father calmly explained that my friend was Roman Catholic and that is what she was instructed. "We were Jews and we do not believe that."

Simple enough as an adult to understand but not a kid. It took me a while to calm down. Just in time years later to see on television a Hasidic mob in New York City bouncing off their collective shoulders a heavily bearded sage by the name of Menachem Mendel Schneerson. An impressive man, leader of the Chabad-Lubavitch spiritual movement who deserved adulation but the group was proclaiming him the Messiah. The Rebbe as he was referred died in 1994. To my discernment there has not yet been an email from the hirsute one. Maybe a fax is forthcoming?

Rabbi Schneur Zalman of Liadi, founder of Schneerson's movement affirmed in the 18th century that "The soul of the Jew is literally part of G-d and Divine essence, while the soul of the Gentile is purely animal in nature even if they are righteous." Sounds like a hater to me! Suffice to say the fundamentalist Hebrew matches up well against their counterparts in Christianity and Islam on the loony scale and if their numbers were larger would probably garner more of the media's attention. Mazel Tov! When the afore-mentioned 12th century philosopher, jurist, and physician Moses Maimonides quipped that the Messiah will come but that "he may tarry," he was perhaps at least ½ right. I think it ends there.

I wondered how many sound-minded young people were made unsound after imbibing the poisons by these consecrated men and women throughout the world. Child abuse in a way. How many nightmares, suicides, psychiatric issues, gender conflicts, prejudices, self-haters, misogynists, etc. produced? If they were so wrong how could billions, some being sensible be affected positively by their sermons?

But popularity does not mean meritorious and history books are replete with naïve majorities and sacrosanct celebrities. Adolph Hitler was "Time Man of the Year" and had many adherents. The isolationist American aviator hero Charles Lindberg gave speeches declaring that a revitalized Nazi Germany must be kept in power or the world order would be decapitated by the expansionist Soviets. A view not surprising for the special guest of Field Marshal

Herman Goering at the 1936 Olympics. Two years later the pilot would proudly wear the Service Cross of the German Eagle given on behalf of the Fuehrer.

Yersinia pestis, the causative agent of the Black Death was wildly popular in the 14th century killing up to 60% of Europe's population. Scientist, not shaman, Alexandre Yersin would isolate the bacteria in 1894 while in Hong Kong.

Some of the most two-faced greedy incompetent doctors and attorneys replete with G-d complexes I have ever met possess the largest unsuspecting client base. Many of the duped unaware are G-d fearing. Perhaps the latter trait helps explain the tragic casuistry.

The incomparable Christopher Hitchens in his book *G-d is not so Great* early on writes that "it (religion) has almost single-handedly warped our attempts at understanding our origins, that it has thrown us into a solipsistic frenzy, that it has repressed our sexuality with particular attention to women, that it has laid the foundation for fantasy-thought processing, and has served as an accomplice to some of the most totalitarian secular regimes."

It seems to me that many oleaginous evangelists of many denominations prey (with an "e") on human fears and hopes based on supernatural premises that present itself as shockingly remote. Furthermore I hold in regard that one can be pious and good without the dogged ceremony and religious label. The "Good Samaritan," who was a pagan is merely one example of a person who did not need the universal laws of physics to be suspended in order to know and more importantly do the right thing. "Doctors without Borders" administer their medicines minus the untoward side effect of conversion. The concepts of the "Golden Rule" and "Turn the Other Cheek" were extant prior to the Common Era. The essence of existence and the existence of essence is so metaphysically complex that sermons pullulated for the masses attempting to explain the distinction would be better served on Comedy Central.

I was aware as the amusement ride now descends, that such scientific luminaries as Sir Isaac Newton, Copernicus, Pasteur, and Galileo were G-d fearing but I wanted to see what scientists of the 21st century thought especially the select group working with our building block DNA.

Enter Francis Collins, head of the National Institutes of Health and previous head of the Human Genome Project. I had of course heard of him but really had no hint about him outside his professional title. He is in one word "remarkable" even if stripped of his Presidential Medal of Honor and National Medal of Science.

Dr. Collins among other things is a physician, geneticist, author, and Evangelical. He has a PhD in physical chemistry from Yale and an M.D. from University of North Carolina. Dr. Rudolf Virchow himself would be impressed. When at Yale he was an atheist but after some soul-searching and being influenced by the magnificent writings of C.S. Lewis he became a believer. He rejects creationism and intellectual design and in 2006 wrote the book *The Language of God: A Scientist Presents Evidence for Belief.*

When the aforementioned Christopher Hitchens who

gave religion no asylum was dying from esophageal cancer it was Dr. Collins he turned to for advice regarding targeted gene therapy to possibly extend his life. Unfortunately with a family history of the same malignancy coupled with years of excess tobacco and alcoholism his neoplasia was out of science's reach.

So a premier scientist in the United States who deals with life at the most basic and complex level not only accepts a divine being but a particular religion along with a plethora of other followers. It does not make the tenets of his creed anymore true but obviously something in his psychology was yearning for spiritual cohesiveness.

Oops there it is! I think that need is in many of us. Perhaps the lure the priest dangled in front of me was beginning to look a little more colorful, more enticing? Dr. Collins is not alone as there are many other prominent scientists sharing the same campfire. To automatically turn a deaf ear serves in my view to blind us from the realm of possibility which in itself is the quiddity and wonderment of science.

I am entrenched in the belief that religious affiliation no matter how transmogrified the product is neither all good nor all bad. Fundamentalism however seems to serve a rather large all- you- can- eat buffet table of bad. How can it not as it is unchained from reason and due to their essentialities the two are born delinked. Anything worth saving is worth attacking and anything worth attacking should survive the imbroglio. After all the faithful have a huge numerical advantage. Quite frankly if religion with all its historical detritus and platitudes were obliterated I think the interstices would predominantly fill with one or more other bad "isms," like rabid nationalism, racism, fascism, unrestrained capitalism, imperialism, corrupt socialism, etc.

If the Bible, Quran, or any sanctified book were to be proven to be 100% palpably false I do not suppose that the Pope or any other religious superstar would hang up their gaudy robes and hop on a motorcycle along with their followers and head to the beach. Infinite spirit and communion may very well be an evolutionary step embedded into the human psyche. There may be a faith-module that is hard-wired within us. It will in my view never be eradicated. Moreover is there anything really wrong that even if it is all total mythology that it gives some in our species hope, that some people may act better, that they may become more charitable, that we are more apt to forgive, that it assuages our pain, and gives us a safe place to moor our restlessness?

Napoleon once stated that "Fiction is for chambermaids," but that is simply not so. Some of the greatest literature along with its important insights and lessons are fictional accounts. Could you imagine any successful 12 step program whether it be for alcoholism or any addiction without belief in some deity? How could Afro-Americans enslaved for centuries in this republic have persisted in their collective sanity without doctrine and church? A mother who loses her child? How much more of European Jewry would have perished in WWII if not for the congregants of the Demark synagogues aiding their escape to neutral Sweden along with good Christians? The Arab Spring was fomented by a multitude of factors, one of them being the liberation theology and demands for social justice raised in Mosques. The white government of South Africa contained many that used the Bible as a lattice to support years of Apartheid, but it was the religious Christian Deputy President F.W. de Klerk who saw it differently. Interpretation being the keyword in religion because interpretative myopia is all too prevalent. However is it righteous to erase belief because of its collisions with the science of the day? The science of tomorrow may be different.

Religious scholar Karen Armstrong feels that belief needs to return to the transformative Axial age. This was the time in our history as envisioned and subsequently coined by German philosopher Karl Jasper when new ways of thinking appeared in Persia, China, India, Greece, Rome, and Judea. This era spanned from the 8th to the 3rd centuries B.C. It included some of the greatest sages such as Confucius, Lao-Tse, Zarathustra, Parsva, Mahavira, Buddha, Isaiah, Elijah, Jerimiah, Homer, Heraclitus, and Plato to name but a few. These prophets were influential in shaping their respective religions and bibles and had a profound effect on the world via the spread of Christianity and secularism. Our Bible with its roots in Canaan is just one of many, a fact frequently ignored or discounted. The Quran which according to Islam is the final revelation from G-d was a still a thousand years away. A revelation that appears a bit plagiarized and doctored up.

It seems to me that the Renaissance and the Enlightenment were natural Axial Age extensions. Armstrong is on the record stating that the Enlightenment was the 2nd Axial Age. Nevertheless our Bible when cherry-picked which is done daily has some amazing commentary but so do other texts. The Sermon on the Mount is worth reading many times over in fact but so is Dostoyevsky and Shakespeare.

Perhaps it would be better for mankind if all the fusty scriptures were allowed to breathe a bit and undergo some syncretism. Diva Tina Turner credits her emotional survival to the disparate alliterative combination of **B**aptism and **B**uddhism. **B.B**. King must be smiling. Rock and Roll Hall of Fame inductee, poet, novelist, songwriter Leonard Cohen uses a mixture of Judaism, Buddhism, and Zen to cope with the raucous universe. There are many who tinker and cobble with the varying philosophies. The Spanish saying *Mestizaje es grandeza* meaning "Mixture is greatness," could not find a more apropos application other than perhaps ethnicity, than in religion. Overall I find that implementation unlikely as extreme territorialism reigns under the penumbra of belief.

Buddhists in general appear to be a more bloodless group not requiring a hematologist with a mop but veneers will always remain just that. Their history is replete with violence and aggression. Documentary evidence of this is found in Japan, Thailand, Myanmar, India, Sri Lanka, and other parts of Southeast Asia. Strict interpretation of verbiages originally written for those in the low-tech wilderness no matter what part of the globe are fraught with tawny rules and approximations covered with layers of verdigris. They are then in unadulterated fashion passed on as pristine purities often aggrandized by disturbed fundamentalists. I suspect the personalities of the original aggrieved scribes and today's zealots are very similar. A dangerous sort no matter the faction or the century.

Nevertheless if the Passover story and the Exodus is a total hoax but families and communities are drawn closer together during the annual Seder should it be expunged simply because of its fiction? Cannot the same be said for Christmas or Easter? Are alternative histories necessarily bad? Maybe "Abe Lincoln: Vampire Hunter" was but not all of them. Are we being intellectually dishonest? The answer in my view must be yes, but most on this planet do not care. Perhaps for us average people it is a small price to pay for what we get back in kind if viewed through an enlightened lens. It is a transaction that I personally can live with hopefully for a long time. I think the old lens grinder and philosopher Spinoza might have agreed. Buddha teaches us that" Life is suffering." If an abstract being helps us endure that suffering should that anodyne be summarily cast away because many of its foundations lied in quicksand?

I always thought that like Voltaire if I was questioned to possibly renounce the Devil on my death bed I would flippantly answer as did he which was "This is no time to make enemies." I am no Voltaire. Perhaps the great French philosopher feared for his élan vital while imprisoned in the Bastille for a year in 1717 but he stuck to his principles to the very end. Interestingly Wolfgang Mozart who was touring Europe at the time was delighted when the godless man passed on. Oh when crazy- in- the- head genius collides outside of Switzerland! I imagine there might be perhaps a day of reckoning, if so we might see on what side of the Maginot line lies the truth. Pascal's cowardly wager (basically you have nothing to lose in believing if it is false and everything to gain if it is true) is alive and well.

After the embolism in 2013 I was petrified. Every time I experienced shortness of breath I was convinced that it was the end. That dyspnea along with fatigue is an ongoing challenge even two years later. All my analysis, all those years of taking care of patients, and my inherent fortitude could not loosen this monster's grip. I have wonderful physicians surrounded by state of the art technology but that does not assuage the angst nor make the breathing easier. When Louis Pasteur's child was dying he wrote in his diary "Science is powerless." I remember that exact feeling under the same circumstances 28 years ago. Two centuries later science is stronger than ever but for many situations it is still powerless.

For every new answer to an old question science generates new questions and so it goes. Given enough time will it provide the answers to the following? Who are we? Why are we here? What is our purpose? What is the ultimate meaning of our existence? What does it mean to be good? Maybe but I tend to doubt it. Science has given us so much but it cannot give us everything. I still do not understand why skin and liver cells regenerate with such ease and auditory hair cells, those functional units responsible for sensorineural hearing do not. I thought evolution mandated that we discern our hidden predators without hearing aids? I am certain some biologist can explain to me that paradox along with the significance of the aforementioned barber's. There are gaps in evolution as previously mentioned.

For me at least with my most recent supplication, blood thinners, follow-up visits, and anti-embolism stockings are all part of my treatment protocol. With apolitical faithfulness there is no steep co-pay and the investment may pay unearthly dividends despite the hypocritical design. Sometimes the absolutely only thing that prevents me from returning in a panic to the emergency room is gratitude to a source I cannot fully explain or just acknowledging to myself that I am no longer required to. With everything that has occurred I feel blessed despite at times appearing as a silhouette of myself. Indeed every man's road to self-actualization is littered with his used and useless ideas along with the new ones. I am of the opinion that they are all recyclable.

I am not alone as study upon study in both the psychological and medical fields present some evidence to suggest that spirituality and belief have a positive impact on a person's well-being. PubMed 2008 research paper 18853749 by Lissoni P, et al concludes: "This preliminary study suggests that spiritual faith may positively influence the efficacy of chemotherapy and the clinical course of neoplastic disease, at least in lung cancer, by improving the lymphocytic-mediated anticancer immune response."

An article appearing April 25th 2013 by psychologist David Rosmarin, et al in The Journal of Affective Disorders entitled "A Test of Faith in God and Treatment" concludes that "Belief in God, but not religious affiliation, was associated with better treatment outcomes. With respect to depression, this relationship was mediated by belief in the credibility of treatment and expectations for treatment gains."

Bookstores are packed with tomes on the subject as faith is gaining popularity in healthcare along with holism as previously mentioned. However when studies are conducted to see if intercession prayer works and is put under the lens of hard science with the same P value (a statistical tool that measures the results observed and the" pure chance" explanation for those results) used in hard science, there has been no proof that it does. Similar experiments have thus far been proven to be a failure. So the undulating thread continues to weave its way through the fabric of the variegated universe.

With that observation and lack of proof every morning I recite the Lord's Prayer and do the same upon retiring. I feel better when I do and I am more open to alternative solutions that are not considered mainstream. If I have surgery scheduled and need to go off blood thinners so I do not hemorrhage on the operating table, I recite it more. One might do much worse. Despite the liberal P-value, my world contains no flying white horses, nor seraphs, nor angels. Quite frankly with all of them purported to have existed in the biblical and Quran narratives there should have been some rather large mid-air collisions. There were after all no computerized traffic control towers or ziggurats during those antiquated times. Perhaps there were accidents and the ad hoc committee did not feel them newsworthy. Perhaps they did but the written record was vanquished by time. Unlikely. I think the only burning bushes that ever existed belonged to the sybaritic concubines of the polytheist-turned monotheist Abraham and his male coevals. Parting seas, multiple resurrections, a swallowing whale, and the rest of the miracles are in my view fatuous not fabulous. There can be I conceive science cohabitating with the glory of G-d. If one does not mind some urban slang, it is the fundamentalist who *ain't* keeping it real or representing.

Some make a pact with the Devil, I made one with G-d but not with his discrepant story-tellers. There is a huge difference in its ramifications. If it all sounds a tad anfractuous, how can it not be? Simmering under every foundation must lie a healthy footer of doubt. I dare say that behind reason there is revelation and behind revelation, there is reason. It is their ratio and not the absolute value of the constants that matter. I cannot imagine a world without either.

Socrates asked "How do you know what you know?" You don't. To me a god and one's relationship with him or her or it is an inner personal representation.

Sam Harris, one of the brilliant "new atheists" to recently emerge has written numerous books on the ills of religion. One of them is entitled "The End of Faith," but authors like Ann Coulter and Bill O'Reilly who predict that without G-d "slavery, genocide, bestiality, anarchy, and crime" will ensue. They will far outsell him. With all due respect to" Annie Get Your Gun" and Billy the Kid O'Really" we have all that with a *Prime Mover* in the equation.

I do not see the end of faith ever being plausible. It is hard enough to quit smoking and there are patches, inhalers, nasal sprays, and prescription pills readily available towards that end. Dr. Harris and his colleagues are engaged in a no-win struggle as the data is beyond comprehension. A 2006 Pew study showed that nearly 80% of all Christians believe in the Second Coming with 20% believing it will happen in their lifetime. 62% of white Protestants (mainline) accept that life evolved over time but only 31% accept natural selection. 65% of white evangelicals hold true that humans have always existed in their present forms. Less than 1/3 of all US Christians accept evolution, the theory endorsed by all major scientific societies. Eastern Orthodox Christians, Muslims, and Orthodox Jews also reject it.

There are some counter-trends developing however. A 2015 Pew study showed that Christians are declining, both as a share of the US population and in total number. In the last eight years American adults identifying with Christian groups have dropped from 78.4% to 70.6%. The total dropping from 178 million to 173 million. Within

Christianity the biggest declines have been in the mainline Protestant tradition and among Catholics. The decline in Christians correspond to a rise in the "nones," those with no religious affiliation. The" nones," atheists, and agnostics now account for 22.8% of the population, up from 16.1% since 2007. America is becoming less Christian and more agnostic and atheistic. These trends may not continue on a straight line and can easily reverse. There is a suggestion that the same phenomenon is happening worldwide.

As long as there are children and parents religion is here to stay. As long as there is poverty, disease, inequality, ignorance, pain, economic and social dislocations all tethered to hopelessness, faith is guaranteed to remain. As long as virtue and vice collide there will always be the perception of a supreme architect. With numerous media outlets, televangelism in particular, the theocratic GOP, and shekels pouring in from the devoted both rich and poor it really would take an Armageddon to end it all. Believers and non-believers would have less heart attacks if they could get along in a tenuous truce. Maybe a little less rhetoric and irritability would improve the dialog although I suspect that will not happen soon. I don't think militant atheists are necessarily moody about a god that exists. I think they are temperamental about the humans who have portrayed him along with the mangled ideas that have followed. Nevertheless rapprochement appears an impossibility.

After all this controversy has been ongoing on for as long as human history existed. Socrates condemnation to drink hemlock and The Nazarene's crucifixion are just two prominent examples of what happens when one questions the prevailing cult buttressed by the State. When the Italian astronomer Galileo Galilei was placed under house arrest in 1633 for the heresy of confirming the heliocentric theory he purportedly muttered "Eppur si muove"-And yet it (earth) moves. We need not whisper and shouting at each other will do us no good. Galileo's peripherally positioned earth would be better served if more people would attempt to make a point rather than trying to drive one (point) home.

Maybe instead of focusing on the hopelessness of eradicating a numinous allegiance we should concentrate more on the hope it provides to so many of us. We are after all just human-at times good, bad, and ugly. It has been stated that science flies us to the moon and religion flies us into buildings. It is not that simple of a binary flight pattern.

We as a species have successfully emerged from the sea but we do "tarry" out from the fog.

As to the important thickness and height of the Madison wall between Church and State, I do not presuppose that there is enough impermeable mortar. We are going to have to live with the diaphanous barricade. The Founding Fathers wanted to demonstrate that our government was not founded on any religion and to ensure religious freedom, not to necessarily protect the government from its influence.

Needless to say the universal argument over credulity

will continue to see-saw upwards and downwards until mankind is no longer available to pullulate a new one, whether it be pro or con.

Probably when the last jackal gets his ass out of the city of Hazor. (Reference Jeremiah 49:33)

CHAPTER: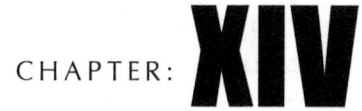

EXODUS
The LAST BREATH,
AN ADMIXTURE OF THINGS

ONE MAY BE surprised to learn that March is the official "Deep Vein Thrombosis Awareness Month" sponsored by the Coalition to Prevent Deep- Vein Thrombosis. David Bloom's former wife Melanie teamed up with Bonnie Bernstein and are leading spokes-persons for the group. This coalition was funded by pharmaceutical company Sanofi-Aventis. I took a shot at trying to contact Ms. Bernstein using her website's email but never heard back. Quite frankly I think all the celebrity *Contact Me* links should have a laugh track music file that plays after you hit "Send." Dr. Gino Merli with whom I had consulted with in the past when I was in clinical medicine is the coalition's physician.

Henry Bussey who cofounded another wonderful organization in 2000 known as Clot Care emailed and alerted me to the actuality that the North American Thrombosis Forum (NATF) will be taking over the Coalition to Prevent Deep-Vein Thrombosis. Clotcare.com is an exquisite website replete with information, testimonials, and videos germane to the topic of VTE. It also has helpful links to other websites. It is a 501(C) 3 non-profit organization that relies on donations. I hope the reader will contribute. This humble author intends to take all the profits from this novella and divide them equally between the aforementioned organizations and The American Foundation for Suicide Prevention.

Bearing a striking verisimilitude to clotcare.com is clotconnect.org which is an information and outreach program sponsored by the University of North Carolina at Chapel Hill. The website states that their mission is to "increase the knowledge of blood clots, clotting disorders, and anticoagulation by providing education and support for healthcare professionals." Although the site was produced to help healthcare professionals by furnishing up to date treatment options, I think patients would also find the information useful.

There are many websites regarding deep vein thrombosis and pulmonary embolism and as mentioned previously the morbidity and mortality statistics are quite varied. I personally like clotcare.com and clotconnect.org because of their navigational ease but the CDC and the American Society of Hematology web pages are worth perusing.

Returning to the 31 days of March, "Deep Vein Thrombosis Awareness Month" was made official by United States Senate Resolution 56 in 2003. It is also "Women's History Month." I would venture to say that most Americans have no sense of either representation. I was a bit crestfallen when my favorite radio-physician pulmonologist Dr. Frank Adams on satellite's "Doctor Radio" had spots lauding the first woman American physician Elizabeth Blackwell during the third month of the year but made no mention about VTE. I was soon relieved on March 25th 2014, the 24 hours before National Cheesesteak Day when he did. Caller after caller kept stating that they had no idea about "DVT Awareness Month" and very little knowledge about the actual disease. Dr. Blackwell, a true pioneer deserves as many spots as allotted but perhaps the producers can mix it up a bit throughout March? I think it is one of the most "unaware" aware months in the United States despite the sentient efforts of rather prodigious medical societies and governmental institutions. Perhaps when the highly publicized NCCA Basketball Tournament known as "March Madness" begins maybe they can highlight this terrible disease. It would be madness not to take this slam- dunk.

It would be an inexcusable breach of prudence not to mention Dr. Charles Gluek from the Jewish Hospital in Cincinnati. His posted article dated August 2013 on clotcare.com entitled "Osteonecrosis, DVT/PE & Central Retinal Vein Thrombosis in Women after Receiving Testosterone" is an interesting read. Lots of big words but no bigger than this man's heart. In the posting there is a statement that says "Dr. Glueck will be glad to provide free assistance in the diagnosis and therapy of women who sustain thrombosis while on testosterone therapy." He invites such women to contact him directly at cjglueck@healthpartners.org.

I can attest that he helps men too. He has emerging data supporting the hypothesis that men even when they are adequately anticoagulated and on testosterone can still have thrombus formation. I must admit when I put my androgen (male hormone) on in the morning, his words become particularly emotive.

When I had my pulmonary embolism I reached out to him and he got back to me immediately. After a few doctor-talk emails he sent me the lab slips needed to check for thrombophilia. I had other questions in the ensuing months and he was there for me, sometimes when nobody else was. Perhaps because they became disinterested. There was indeed an inexpressible yet palpable concern from miles away. He also followed up to see how I was doing. His last sentence in his last email to me was "Get the word out." I promised him that I would. The Lord knows I have made every effort to keep my word and ring the tocsin once more. It is the very least I can do for a gentleman who has had a most salutary influence on my life.

We need to put out an Amber Alert for DVT/PE. This disease is missing from our stream of consciousness and is unfortunately in this case alive and well. It is my hope that I accomplished that which I had set out to do which was to illustrate from lamb to loom how this fiend is created, its lair, what highways it moves on, and the damage this creature creates.

I suspect I must suspend my most wished hopeful accomplishment until both the public and medical community catch on and the intellectual currency increases in value. It is time for the Gordian knot to be finally cut. I

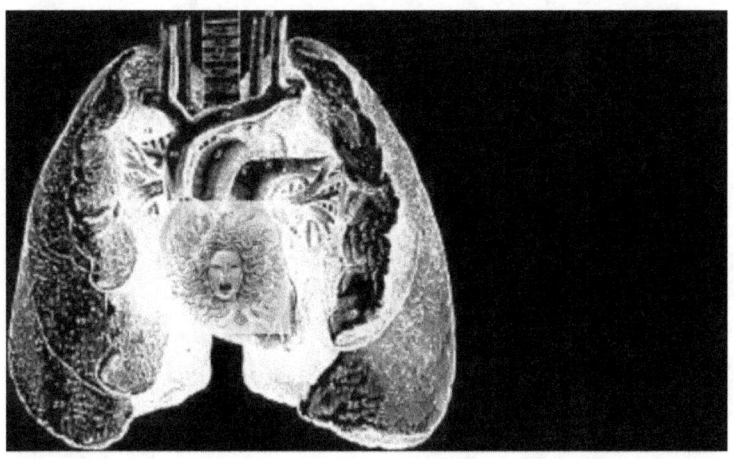

believe I have made a strong case, I hope I have not been a weak and feckless advocate.

Like the previous blood-letting physicians that paved the way, we continue to scratch the surface. I think we always will in the practice of medicine. Nevertheless for now the disease needs to be placed front and center in our medical mindfulness and remain. If not it will continue to "glut the maw of death" as monsters often do after they are done terrorizing their captives in a cauldron.

As long as blood courses through our veins there will always be disease. The universe is so made that it cannot be without. Our best and only defense against these Medusa-like illnesses are the pleuropotential seeds of technology sowed in the ever expanding arable field of knowledge and the fruits that are harvested. Unlike" The "Apple" in Genesis the vintage crop should be incessantly bitten into and thoroughly digested. Over and over again as curiosity needs to be encouraged and not the opposite.

Indeed the ultimate solutions to life's multifaceted puzzles often involves the previous referenced "A combination of things."

BIBLIOGRAPHY

AARP Bulletin. Peterson Johnathan. Securing the Future 07/2015

Allen Brooke. Moral Minority Our Skeptical Founding Fathers 2006

American Family Physician.com Deep Vein Thrombosis and Pulmonary Embolism 05/08/2015

AnticoagulationHUB.com. Richard Pizzi. CDC to Celebrate Blood Clot Strategies
11/04/2015

Arendt Hannah. The Origins of Totalitarianism 1951

Armstrong Karen. The Battle for God 2000

Armstrong Karen. The Bible 2007

Armstrong Karen. The Great Transformation 2007

Armstrong Karen. The Case for God 2010

Ascher Abraham. Russia 2002

Aslan Reza. Zealot 2013

Barlow Nora. The Autobiography of Charles Darwin 1958

Bleacherreport.com. Carroll Will. Perils of Blood Clot

End Season for Cavs' Anderson Varejao

Cdc.gov. Data and Statistics. DVT/PE. 06/22/2015

Cdc.gov. Reyes Nimia, Grosse Scott, Grant Althea. Deep Vein Thrombosis & Pulmonary Embolism

Clay Catherine. King Kaiser Tsar 2006

Clevelandclinicmeded.com. Thacker Holly. Hormone Therapy and Risk of Venous Thromboembolism

Clinics in Chest Medicine Stein Paul, M.D. & Fadi Matta M.D. Epidemiology and Incidence: The Scope of the Problem and Risk Factors for Development of VTE. 12/2010

Clotspot.com. What is a Pulmonary Embolism?

Crean Thomas. God is No Delusion: A Refutation of Richard Dawkins 2007

Chatterjee M.D., Saurav, et al. Thrombolysis for Pulmonary Embolism. JAMA 2014

Dawkins Richard. The God Delusion 2006

Dawkins Richard. The Blind Watchmaker 1987

Dawkins Richard. The Greatest Show on Earth: The Evidence for Evolution 2009

Dawkins Richard. An Appetite for Wonder 2013

Danforth John. Faith and Politics 2006

Daniel, D. Prevention of Air Travel Fatalities. 2013

Ellis, Joseph J. American Sphinx: The Character of Thomas Jefferson 1996

Emedicinehealth.com. Pulmonary Embolism: Treatment Guidelines 2014

Escardio.org. Acute Pulmonary Embolism: Diagnosis and Management

European Heart Journal. Konstantaninides, Stavros et al. 2014 Guidelines on Diagnosis and Management of Pulmonary Embolism. 11/14/2014

Everydayhealth.com. Brown Jennifer Phd. How Brian Vickers Overcame DVT and Got Back to Racing

Everydayhealth.com. Rodriguez Diana. 9 Celebrities Who Battled Deep Vein Thrombosis

Fpnotebook.com. Pulmonary Embolism

Circulation Goldhaber M.D. &C. Elliot M.D.: Acute Pulmonary Embolism. 12/2003

Hahn Scott, Wiker Benjamin. Answering the New Atheism: Dismantling Dawkins' Case against God 2008

Harris Sam. The Moral Landscape How Science Can Determine Human Values 2010

Harris Sam. The End of Faith Religion Terror and the Future of Reason 2004

Harris Sam. Waking Up: A Guide to Spirituality without Religion 2014

Hawking Stephen, Mlodinow L. The Grand Design 2010

Hawking Stephen. A Brief History of Time: From the Big Bang to Black Holes 1988

Hitchens Christopher. God is not Great How Religion Poisons Everything 2007

Hitchens Christopher. Christopher Hitchens and His Critics Terror, Iraq, and the Left 2008

House Adrian. Francis of Assisi 2000

Haykal, Husayn Muhammad. The Life of Muhammed 1976

Healthline.com. Krans Brian. Pulmonary Embolism. 08/02/2012

House, Adrian. Francis of Assisi 2000

JAMA 2015. Couturaud Francis MD, PhD et al. Six Months vs Extended Oral Anticoagulation after a First Episode of Pulmonary Embolism. The PADIS-PE Randomized Clinical Trial

JAMA 2015. Jiemin Ma, PhD, MHS et al. Temporal Trends in Mortality in the United States, 1969-2013

Jewish Publication Society, Berlin Adele, Brettler Marc Zvi, et al. The Jewish Study Bible 1985

Kelchner, Wesley John. The Bible and King Solomon's Temple in Masonry 1924

Krauss, Lawrence M. A Universe from Nothing 2013

Levitin, D. The Organized Mind: Thinking Straight in the Age of Information Overload 2014

Lissoni, P, et al. Pub Med 18853749. 2008

Lung.org. Understanding Pulmonary Vascular Disease.

Mayo Clinic.com Pulmonary Embolism: Take Measures to lower your risk

MedicineNet.com. Deep Vein Thrombosis and Pulmonary Embolism

Medscape Pulmonary Embolism: Practice Essentials, Background, Anatomy 2015

Merckmanuals.com. Pulmonary Embolism

Mlodinow Leonard. Euclid's Window 2001

Mlodinow Leonard. The Drunkard's Walk: How Randomness Rules Our Lives 2008

Nadler Steven. Spinoza A Life 1999

National Blood Clot Alliance.com. Pulmonary Embolism

National Institutes of Health MedlinePlus.com Pulmonary Embolism

Oberman, Heiko A. Luther: Man between God and the Devil 2006

Office of the Surgeon General United States. The Surgeon General's Call to Action to Prevent Deep Vein Thrombosis and Pulmonary Embolism 2008.

PulmCCM.org. Pulmonary Embolism

Papadakis, Maxine, Mcphee Stephen, Rabow Michael, ed. Current Medical Diagnosis & Treatment 2016

Radiopaedia.org. D'Souza, Donna et al. Pulmonary Embolism/Radiology Reference Article

Radzinsky Edvard. The Last Tsar 1992

Rosmarin, D, et al. Journal of Affective Disorders. Test of Faith in God and Treatment

Ross Steward. The Israeli-Palestinian Conflict 2007

Russel Bertrand. Why I am not a Christian 1957

Russel Bertrand. Wisdom of the West 1977

Science Daily.com Pulmonary Embolism

Simms Brendan. Europe 2014

Slate.com Orfri Danielle. The Tyranny of Perfection. 9/25/2014

Spellberg Denise A. Thomas Jefferson's Qur'an: Islam and the Founders 2013

Spong, John Shelby. Rescuing the Bible from Fundamentalism 1991

Stanfordhealthcare.org. Pulmonary Embolism

Stenger Victor. God the Failed Hypothesis 2008
Stenger Victor. The New Atheism 2009
Stenger Victor. God and the Multiverse 2014
Thrombosisadviser.com. Pulmonary Embolism
Vascularweb.org. Pulmonary Embolism
WebMD.com Pulmonary Embolism: Topic Review
Wikipedia.com